The Thrust Plate Hip Prosthesis

Springer
Berlin
Heidelberg
New York
Barcelona
Budapest
Hong Kong
London
Milan
Paris
Santa Clara
Singapore
Tokyo

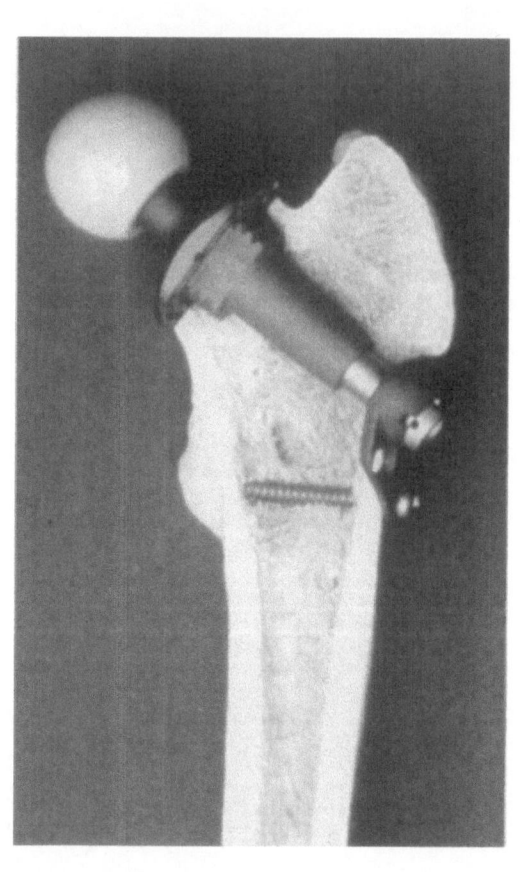

A.H. Huggler   H.A.C. Jacob   (Eds.)

The Thrust Plate Hip Prosthesis

With 96 Figures, Some in Colour, and 5 Tables

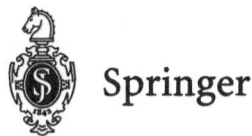 Springer

ARNOLD H. HUGGLER, M.D.
Orthopaedic Department
Canton Hospital
Loestrasse 170
7000 Chur
Switzerland

HILAIRE A.C. JACOB, Ph.D.
Biomechanic Unit
Department of Orthopaedic Surgery Balgrist
University of Zürich
Forchstrasse 348
8008 Zürich
Switzerland

ISBN-13: 978-3-642-64433-7   e-ISBN-13: 978-3-642-60502-4
DOI: 10.1007/978-3-642-60502-4

Library of Congress Cataloging-in-Publication Data. The thrust plate hip prosthesis/A.H. Huggler, H.A.C. Jacob (eds.).   p.   cm. Based on an international symposium held in Zurich in 1994. Includes bibliographical references and index. ISBN-13: 978-3-642-64433-7 (Hardcover:alk. paper) 1. Artificial hip joints – Congresses. I. Huggler, Arnold H. II. Jacob, Hilaire A.C. [DNLM: 1. Hip Prosthesis – congresses. 2. HIP Joint-surgery – congresses. WE 860 T531 1997] RD549. T537 1997 617.5'810592–dc20 DNLM/DLC for Library of Congress 96-34374

© Springer-Verlag Berlin Heidelberg 1997
Softcover reprint of the hardcover 1st edition 1997

The use of general descriptive names, registered names, trademarks, etc. in this publication does not imply, even in the absence of a specific statement, that such names are exempt from the relevant protective laws and regulations and therefore free for general use.

Product Liability: The publishers cannot guarantee the accuracy of any information about dosage and application contained in this book. In every individual case the user must check such information by consulting the relevant literature.

Cover design: Design & Production GmbH, Heidelberg

Typesetting: Scientific Publishing Services (P) Ltd, Madras

SPIN: 10465325   24/3135/SPS – 5 4 3 2 1 0 – Printed on acid-free paper

Preface

As is probably the case with all successful innovations, the unique design of the thrust plate prosthesis (TPP) was not born of a sudden fancy for a radically different hip joint replacement, but emerged from elaborate biomechanical investigations on the loosening of conventional, intramedullarly anchored hip prosthesis shafts.

In the 1970s, hip revisions due to loosening of the prostheses became a burden to patients not only physically and psychologically but also economically. This meant that it also became a matter of daily concern to the orthopaedic surgeon, who then had to cope with new, previously unknown problems. Loosening processes were detected within 5 years of implantation in up to 25% of cases. While implant loosenings were considered to be the result of incorrect handling of materials, we felt that a number of details still had to be considered in regard to the behavior of the entire bone–prosthesis complex and the action of mechanical forces.

Our initial step in developing the TPP was therefore based both on long-term clinical experience with hip prostheses and also on the results of experimental stress analyses. These drew our attention to the unphysiological manner in which the bone is loaded by intramedullarly anchored prostheses. Here we were guided by the observations of Hermann von Meyer (1815–1892), Karl Culmann (1821–1881), and Julius Wolff (1836–1902), who were the first to observe the relationship between the architecture of bone and the mechanical forces that act on the bone structure, and were also led by the findings of Friedrich Pauwels (1885–1980). We designed a prosthesis that transmits the hip force to the bone in a more physiological manner by means of a thrust plate placed on the resected neck of the femur.

Hey Groves (1922), Wiles (1938), the brothers Robert and Jean Judet (1946), McKee (1950), and Picchio (1957) among others, introduced cementless prostheses which were attached to the femur without intramedullary fixation. These prostheses may show some similarities to the TPP at a quick glance, but they differ basically from it in that they do not take into account the specific function of the cortical bone at the proximal end of the femur. Also, the materials used could not fulfill all the requirements demanded.

When we first conceived the TPP in 1976, manufacturers showed little interest in it. Neither the first prototypes made for experimental testing nor the two prototypes of the TPP subjected to clinical trial in Chur in 1978 would have been possible without the active support provided by Mr. Hermann Straehl and Mr. Max Briner of Sulzer Brothers Ltd.

Through Prof. Adam Schreiber (former Chairman of the Department of Orthopaedic Surgery, Balgrist, University of Zurich), the Ida-Herzog-Egli Foundation raised the required funds in 1980 to manufacture the first limited series of prostheses, 64 of which were implanted between 1980 and 1985. This pilot study was a joint venture with the Department of Orthopaedic Surgery, Balgrist, University of Zurich, following approval by the ethical commission of the Balgrist hospital, allowing initially 20 prostheses to be implanted. The remaining 44 were implanted in the Orthopaedic Department of the Canton Hospital in Chur. Since we were dealing with an unconventional new hip prosthesis, it was especially beneficial that the Orthopaedic University Clinic was participating in the pilot field study. This was important not only to confirm that the TPP can be a preferable alternative to the conventional hip prostheses but especially to identify possible weaknesses of the prosthesis with the assistance of a second authority. We are very grateful to Prof. Adam Schreiber for this collaboration.

We are very indebted to Mr. André Buchel, Director of Sulzer Medica, Dr. Walter Kaiser (former Director of Allo Pro Ltd.), and Mr. Erwin Locher, Director of Allo Pro Ltd., who supported this project. We express our appreciation as well to Mr. Hans-Ruedi Lötscher (former Director of Allo Pro Ltd.) who encouraged us in the early developmental stages.

We are also indebted to all those from Allo Pro Ltd. and Sulzer Medical Technology Ltd. who contributed with their valuable help in realizing this project.

We are particularly obligated to Mr. Urs Lack and Dr. Martin Schmidt of Allo Pro Ltd. (now Sulzer Orthopedics) and to Springer-Verlag for the competent management which made this monograph possible.

The favourable clinical results of the TPP which we obtained together with the Orthopaedic University Clinic Balgrist, has further strengthened our firm belief in this concept. It also led us to include other orthopaedic specialists in an extended field study to gain a wider range of experience before presenting the TPP to a still larger orthopaedic community. This presentation took place at an international symposium held in Zurich in 1994, organized by Allo Pro Ltd., at the Orthopaedic University Clinic Balgrist, which extended its hospitality to all the participants.

We know of no other prosthesis which has been evaluated clinically for more than 12 years before being released for general use.

The symposium in Zurich encouraged us to publish the personal contributions of the participants and to relate our experiences in detail. This volume provides the opportunity to present individual viewpoints both by the orthopaedic surgeons who first carried the TPP into the clinical field and by the manufacturers whose interest has been expressed in this prosthesis. Throughout these years they have contributed valuable suggestions toward materializing the clinical use of the TPP and in the design of the implantation instruments, which are almost as important as the implant itself.

To guarantee its reliability, a great number of details must be considered meticulously regarding the clinical feasibility and technical quality of the TPP. The increasing demand for the TPP confirms its value, and we are therefore not surprised to see a growing number of imitators. While imitation may be interpreted positively, one must recognize that the imitations themselves do not necessarily reflect the potential of experience built into the original; neither do they display the same quality of material, which is an absolute prerequisite.

The viewpoints and opinions expressed in the contributions presented here are those of the respective authors. They do not necessarily reflect the opinions of the editors or the publishers.

Maienfeld   ARNOLD H. HUGGLER
Winterthur   HILAIRE A.C. JACOB
May 1996

Contents

List of Contributors

ABAD RICO, J.I.
Hospital Regional Carlos Haya, Avda. de Carlos Haya,
29106 Malaga, Spain

BEREITER, H.
Rhätisches Kantonsspital, Loestraße 170, 7000 Chur, Switzerland

BÜRGI, M.
Abteilung für Biomechanik, Sulzer Orthopädie,
8400 Winterthur, Switzerland

FINK, B.
Heinrich-Heine-Universität, Moorenstraße 5, 40001 Düsseldorf,
Germany

GRUBER, G.
Orthop. Universitätsklinik, Paul-Meimbergstraße 3, 35385 Gießen,
Germany

HAUSER, R.
Spital Neumünster, Trichtenhauserstrasse 12, 8125 Zollikerberg,
Switzerland

HUGGLER, A.H.
Rhätisches Kantonsspital, Loestraße 170, 7000 Chur, Switzerland

JACOB, H.A.C.
Orthopädische Universitätsklinik Balgrist, Forchstrasse 340,
8008 Zürich, Switzerland

KERN, S.
Spital Limmattal, Urdorferstrasse 100, 8952 Schlieren,
Switzerland

KORNELY, E.
Heinrich-Heine-Universität, Moorenstraße 5, 40001 Düsseldorf,
Germany

KUHN, T.
Kantonsspital Uri, Spitalplatz, 6460 Altdorf, Switzerland

MENGE, M.
St. Marienkrankenhaus, Salzburgerstrasse 15, 67067 Ludwigshafen,
Germany

RÜTHER, W.
Orthopädische Klinik, Univ.-Krankenhaus Eppendorf,
Martinistraße 52, 20246 Hamburg, Germany

SCHENK, R.K.
Pathophysiologisches Institut, Universität Bern, Murtenstraße 35,
3010 Bern, Switzerland

SCHMIDT, M.
Sulzer Orthopedics Ltd., 6341 Baar, Switzerland

SCHNEIDER, T.
Heinrich-Heine-Universität, Moorenstraße 5, 40001 Düsseldorf,
Germany

SCHWARZENBACH, U.
Orthopädische Chirurgie, Volkshausstrasse 20, 9630 Wattwil,
Switzerland

STREICHER, R.M.
Wingertlistrasse 12, 8405 Winterthur, Switzerland

STÜRZ, H.
Orthop. Universitätsklinik, Paul-Meimbergstraße 3, 35385 Gießen,
Germany

CHAPTER 1

The Thrust Plate Prosthesis:
A New Experience in Hip Surgery

A.H. HUGGLER

History of Hip Endoprosthetics

Prosthesis Loosening

Until the end of the 1950s, the possibilities of surgically treating painful, crippling hip conditions were restricted to arthrodeses and operations of the Girdlestone and Milch Batchelor type. General implant surgery, and hip endoprosthetics in particular, began to develop rapidly. Endoprostheses fixed to the proximal end of the femur were considered to be a decisive step forward compared to the earlier methods of treatment, and a breakthrough in the history of modern orthopaedic surgery. Good mid-term results with intramedullarly fixed femoral prostheses led to an unshakeable belief in this system. A few alternative procedures did not achieve the same measure of success.

Unfortunately, long-term results were not always as good. This is reflected by the number of revision operations as a result of prosthesis loosening which have become a significant portion of daily surgical hip interventions and have also become main themes at orthopaedic congresses.

In the 1970s, revision surgery that became necessary due to infections, cement damage and tissue reactions to wear particles from the articulating surfaces started to become a dramatic challenge because of the elaborate surgical and technical requirements [29]. The requirements on implant materials, materials which were not originally developed for artificial hip joints, could only be partially met at that time. Articulating surfaces manufactured from synthetic materials occasionally led to wear particles and, subsequently, to undesirable tissue reactions. Large loss of osseous tissue in the environment of the implant made stable fixation during revisions, generally done with a larger implant, more difficult. Special revision prostheses for the acetabulum and femur therefore had to be developed. Hip revisions led to physical, psychological and, last but not least, financial burdens for the patient.

Although the rate of loosening was reduced by the introduction of cleanroom technology, improved cementation procedures and better material combinations for articulation, the question of the biomechanical causes of implant loosening remained for the most part unanswered. It was therefore our intention to investigate this question clinically.

In most cases, radiographs of prostheses with intramedullary fixation showed atrophy of the proximal surrounding bone, transformation of the cortex into cancellous bone and thickening of the cortical bone in the distal third of the prosthesis. This structural remodelling has been interpreted as an attempt of the host bone to adapt to the rigid implant. In 1971, Jackson-Burrows [10] reported similar observations on femora fitted with endoprostheses. It remained questionable whether the bone could withstand the forces imposed on it by the prosthesis.

Preoperative observations and radiological follow-up examinations, together with long-term results reported in the literature, reflect the obvious biomechanical nature of these loosening problems. Good long-term results with patients over 65 years of age can be attributed to reduced physical activity [20, 31]. For patients under 50 years of age, unsatisfactory results 10 years after the operation are reported in over 30% of cases [1, 3]. These results are for standard hip prostheses with intramedullary fixation. The bone remodelling process, which depends on functional loading, is obviously unable to provide adequate fixation for the implant.

During endoprosthetic revision operations, it is often noticed that elderly patients seldom exhibit a normal cancellous bone structure in the proximal metaphysis. The poor cancellous bone structure was clearly unable to transmit the load without damage and probably suffered fatigue fracture. We therefore assumed that this would permit a prosthesis with intramedullary fixation to move relative to the surrounding bone, leading to bone resorption and consequent loosening.

Retrospective Observations on Innovative Models of the 1970s and 1980s

In an attempt to master the unresolved biomechanical problems of hip prostheses with intramedullary fixation, some of the more intrepid orthopaedic surgeons set off in two opposite directions, each considered at the end of the 1960s as being a breakthrough:

1. Resurfacing as a method of preserving bone [4, 5, 26, 27], however, turned out to be unsuccessful due to the metal femoral cup that impaired the trophic activity of the femoral head through stress shielding. High peak stresses at the transition to the femoral neck added to the deleterious results [9, 24].
2. Long-stem prostheses by Lord [16] and Judet [15] were also unsuccessful. Suitable load transfer over a large bone surface area had been expected with a long stem, but neither of these prostheses were able to achieve a compromise between proximal and distal load transfer.

Problems with Intramedullarly Anchored Prostheses

Provided the bone cement exhibits a lower modulus of elasticity than the bone and the implant, it might provide suitable load transfer in certain situations. Nevertheless, a rigid prosthesis with intramedullary fixation usually displays unsuitable biomechanical characteristics.

Although the intervening layer of cement improves the form fit of the prosthesis in the bone, high transverse stress peaks still appear locally in proximal–medial and distal–lateral areas. The wedge form of the prosthesis stem additionally leads to circumferential stresses in the cortical bone.

The shape, internal architecture and strength of the proximal end of the femur are a reflection of Wolff's law [30]. The unphysiological architecture of bone that appears as a reaction to prostheses with intramedullary fixation led us to investigate the stresses in the femur experimentally [11, 12].

The dramatic evidence of a 60% reduced loading of the proximal end of the femur compared with normal physiological conditions was most convincing. The cortical bone plays the same role as the pier of a bridge. Where this important load-carrying structure is disturbed by the implanted femoral stem, the familiar loosening problems occur.

The extent of stress shielding producing this unsatisfactory situation in the proximal femur was determined in an analogous manner to previous investigations on the loading of cortical bone in the area of the acetabulum by Jacob et al. in 1976 [13].

Concept

Our efforts were therefore directed towards finding an implant which would, for the most part, preserve the physiological load pattern by a corresponding load transfer, while avoiding intramedullary fixation. After Scholten [23] had independently confirmed our experimental results using finite element analysis, we were encouraged to attempt transmission of the hip load directly to the medial cortical bone of the femoral neck as is physiologically the case.

The thrust plate prosthesis (TPP) was designed in 1976 with the objective of maintaining the magnitude and direction of the physiological stress distribution in the femur. It has been reported in the literature several times since its first clinical use in 1978 [7, 8, 25] and is treated in detail in the chapter by Jacob (see Chap. 2, this volume).

The TPP differs in shape and construction from conventional prostheses. The thrust plate rests on the stump of the femoral neck and, prior to the 1992 version, had a central opening for a mandrel, on which the prosthetic femoral head is mounted. Laterally, this stiff mandrel is firmly anchored with a single bolt to a lateral plate, which itself is fixed to the femur below the tuberculum innominatum by means of two cortical screws. The high bending rigidity of the mandrel and the central bolt ensures firm seating of the thrust plate on the stump of the femoral neck while walking. The initial pre-stressing of the bolt, which presses the thrust plate against the stump of the femoral neck, ensures stable fixation immediately postoperatively. Relaxation of this pre-stressing takes place over several months until a condition of equilibrium sets in [21]. Initially, bone cement was used for the transverse stabilization of the thrust plate in the two 1978 prototypes. With the TPP of the first series in 1980, the surface of the thrust plate in contact with the bone was given a coarse structure, so that locking with the bone occurred, avoiding transverse slip and making cement superfluous (Fig. 1).

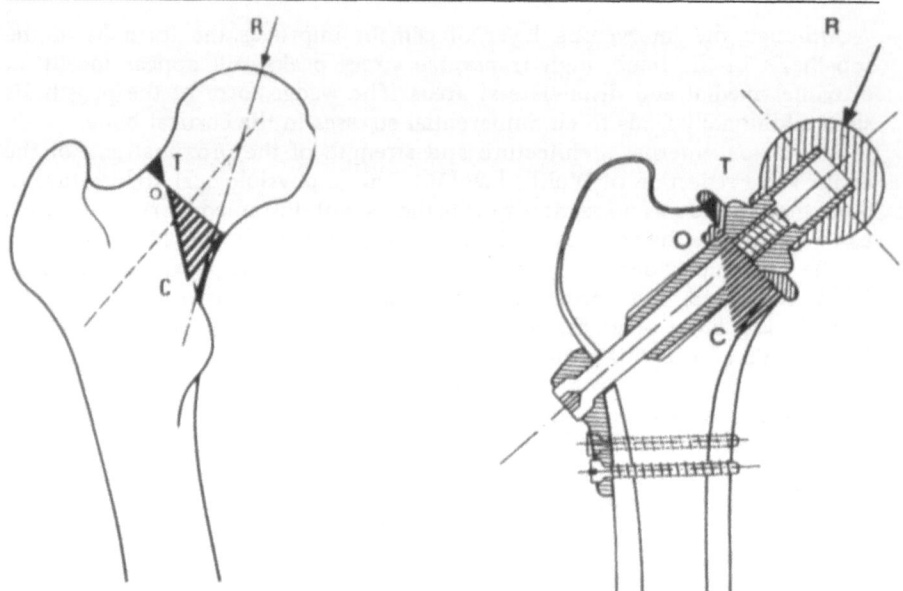

Fig. 1a,b. The physiological compressive (*C, shaded*) and tensile (*T, black*) stresses in the femoral neck are retained following implantation of the thrust plate prosthesis (TPP). *R*, hip joint force

The concept has not changed since the first TPP implantation in 1978 in Chur. The TPP was initially manufactured from a cast cobalt-chromium based alloy, while the bolt was made of forged material. In the first series (1980–1987), the thrust plate was round for economic reasons. It was made oval in the second series (1988–1991) to match the cross-section of the femoral neck. From the second series onwards, titanium has been used for parts seated onto the bone (thrust plate and lateral plate). The particular characteristic of the third and latest series (since 1992) is the fact that the mandrel and thrust plate have been combined into one piece.

The preliminary investigations regarding the basic concept of the TPP, which included behaviour of the bone in the environment of the thrust plate, stress analysis and material testing of the prosthesis components, and the manufacture of surgical instruments required for implantation, were carried out from 1976 to 1978.

After testing all the instruments and the working steps needed for the operation on autopsy specimens, our first two patients were operated on in 1978 in the Canton's Hospital in Chur (Switzerland). Four prototypes of the TPP were available to us for the investigations and the first two operations. A further number of TPP were made available for clinical investigation in September 1980, when the manufacturers were persuaded by the Orthopaedic Department of the University of Zurich, Balgrist (Prof. Dr. med. Adam Schreiber) to produce a small series. After the clinic had granted permission on the basis of the results of our preliminary investigations, 20 TPP were implanted in Zurich and 44 in Chur.

The prospective randomized joint field study was designed to show whether the TPP would meet the above mentioned biomechanical requirements. It was therefore particularly important to study early failures and to determine possible late complications in order to identify the causes and make corresponding corrections.

The strongly protruding boss of the lateral plate in the first series led to local discomfort due to bursitis in some slender male patients. Since the lateral plate was reduced in size in the second and third series of the TPP, there have been no more reports of problems of this nature (Fig. 2).

Following a careful evaluation of the clinical validity of the TPP over a period of more than 10 years at the Orthopaedic/Traumatology Department at the Canton Hospital in Chur and the Balgrist Orthopaedic University Clinic in Zurich, with satisfactory mid-term results, it was then possible, with the assistance of the manufacturers, to extend the TPP test project to other clinics. In 1994, an international exchange of clinical experience with the TPP took place at the Balgrist Orthopaedic University Clinic in Zurich.

Comparison of the Thrust Plate Prosthesis with Other Hip Prostheses with Metaphyseal Fixation

During the development of the TPP, we reviewed the literature available to us concerning hip prostheses with metaphysial fixation from the 1940s and 1950s [2, 6, 14, 17, 22, 28, 32]. The Gambier and Ricchiardi prosthesis remained experimental. Picchio apparently operated on only two patients (1957, 1959 [22]). Results obtained by Zanoli, Wiles and Bonola were also restricted to a few clinical cases.

The femoral prosthesis of the Judet brothers led in a new direction, away from the interposition arthroplastic types such as the Smith-Petersen Cup, in that it was an implant which did not move relative to the bone. In both models, the bone support for the femoral prosthesis was provided by the predominantly cancellous proximal area of the femoral neck, where there is practically no functional cortical bone. This Judet femoral prosthesis had been designed with the intention of preserving the femoral neck. It must be borne in mind that the less the femoral neck is resected, the lower the bending stresses in the prosthesis. On the other hand, with high femoral neck resection, the cortical bone is very thin compared with the femoral calcar lower down.

The Judet prosthesis was modified by various authors by altering the shape of the shaft, for example by using a screw (e.g. [2, 32]) or a nail [19]. These prostheses with metaphysial fixation in the femoral neck and in the trochanter region were different from the diaphysial types, in which there always was an intramedullary stem (albeit short).

Most of these prostheses with metaphysial fixation had a head geometry of little more than a hemisphere and, as in the case of the Judet prosthesis, were anchored in the predominantly cancellous bone in the most proximal area of the femoral neck.

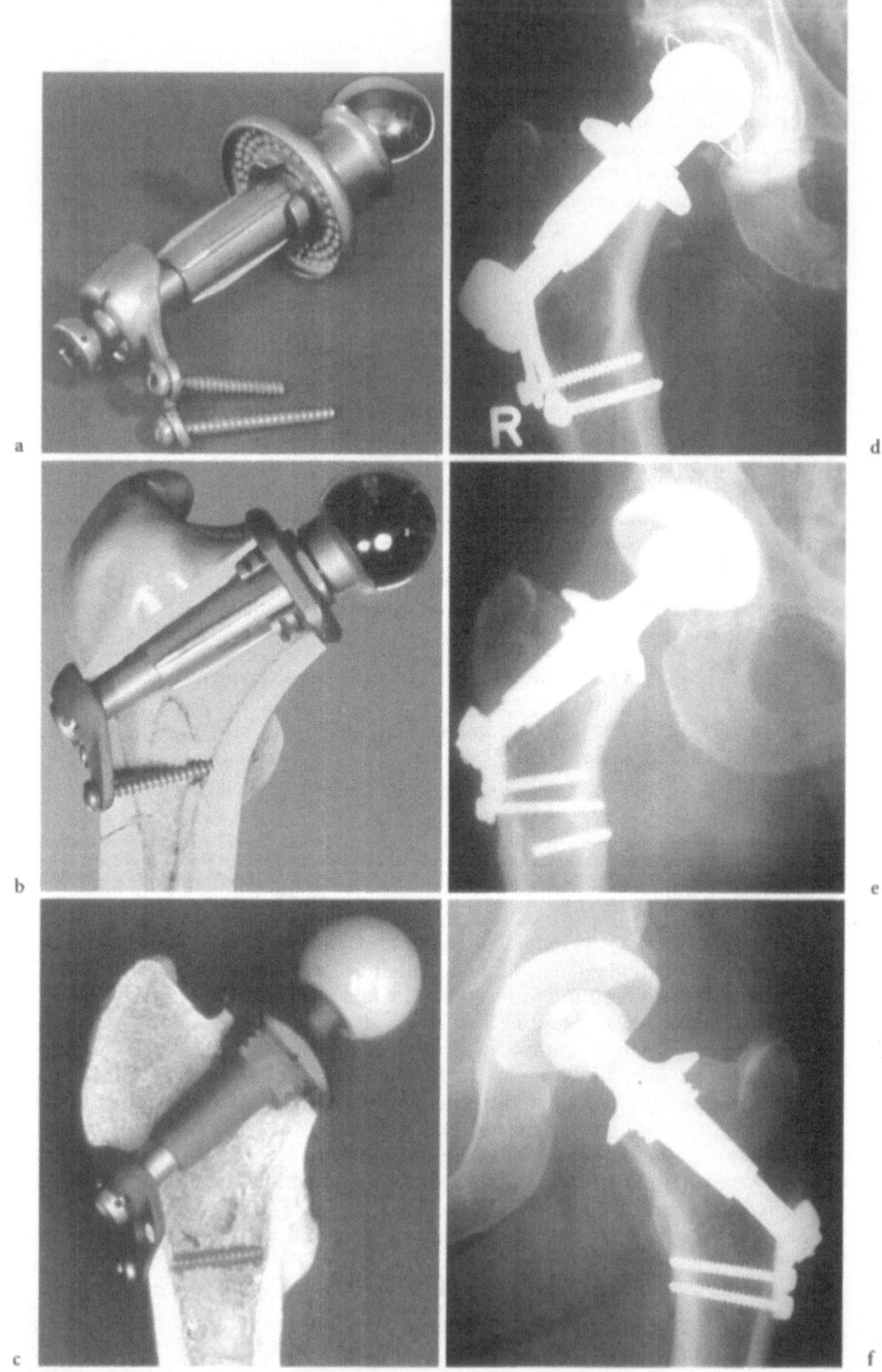

a

b

c

d

e

f

There is therefore, at the most, only an optical similarity between the TPP and the Judet prosthesis.

Areas of Application of the Thrust Plate Prosthesis

Indications

If a total hip endoprosthesis is indicated for a hip disorder, the most suitable implant must first be determined. The selection of a TPP depends on certain additional criteria (see also "Preoperative Planning"): With respect to the anatomy (shape, size, relationship of axes), and bone trophic activity (e.g. necrosis, dystrophy), the proximal end of the femur must permit correct implantation of the TPP. An extremely large or small hip joint with strong anteversion of the femoral neck combined with varus or valgus deformities and a dysplastic acetabulum often requires reconstructive correction measures with custom-made endoprostheses. Although the TPP is well adapted to the structures of the hip joint normally present, its use might not be appropriate where reconstructive corrective measures are needed.

The TPP is as suitable for use in older operable patients as most other conventional implants. If a healthy older patient has a long life expectancy and might even be expected to resume regular physical or even sporting activities, subsequent loosening must be considered if a femoral prosthesis with intramedullary fixation is selected. The use of a TPP is the preferred choice for the primary operation in such a case. For older patients, however, whose life expectancy and physical activity following the operation are assessed as low, there are no compelling reasons for using a TPP, because a satisfactory result can also be expected from a femoral stem prosthesis with intramedullary fixation.

Our oldest patient was 78 years of age at the time of operation. After the operation, she was able to resume work in her own mountain farm until she died 8 years later. Our youngest patient, suffering from disabling juvenile rheumatoid arthritis, was operated on when she was 19 years old.

The indications for a TPP are basically the same as for conventional total hip endoprosthesis; however, there are additional criteria for the implantation of a TPP. It might be stated that a TPP can be used in all hip conditions where the femoral neck exhibits strong medial cortical bone. In addition, the cortical bone

---

Fig. 2a–f. The thrust plate prosthesis (TPP) of the first, second and third series with corresponding radiological follow-up examinations. a First series. b Second series. c Third series. d Female patient born in 1930. Radiograph taken on 2 July 1991, 6 years after implantation of a TPP (first series). The cemented polyethylene cup has begun to wear out, but the TPP is still stable. e Same patient as in Fig. 2d. A revision of the worn-out polyethylene cup became necessary, and it was replaced by a cementless "press-fit" cup. On this occasion, the first-series TPP was exchanged for a second-series TPP. The radiograph was taken 2 years and 9 months postoperatively. f A female patient born in 1920. The radiograph was taken on 19 April 1994, 2½ years after the implantation of a third-series TPP in combination with a cementless "press-fit" cup

must be intact below the tuberculum innominatum. Joint replacement using the TPP can also be recommended for primary and secondary coxarthrosis. Secondary coxarthrosis as a result of a congenital pathological deformity or as a result of growth disturbances is also an appropriate indication, as is arthrosis following hip-joint trauma and rheumatic or bacterial coxitis. Particularly in younger patients, the TPP is a valuable alternative to surgical techniques such as intertrochanteric osteotomy or a conventional standard prosthesis. Biologically elderly patients are probably not suitable for either intertrochanteric osteotomy or for a TPP. Conventional endoprosthetic treatment methods are available for such patients, because, as a rule, patients with a limited life expectancy may not be expected to have daily activities involving major loading of the hip. Intertrochanteric osteotomy is considered a suitable procedure for secondary, but not for primary arthrosis. From experience, the prognosis for intertrochanteric osteotomy in younger patients with secondary coxarthrosis remains uncertain, even with apparently favourable indications. In such patients, we therefore recommend implantation of a TPP from the beginning. It should also be considered that, in the event of an unsatisfactory corrective osteotomy, further treatment often involves inability to work for over 1 year. Motivation for the necessary second intervention can scarcely be expected.

Femoral head necrosis requires special attention. As a rule, femoral head necrosis begins segmentally, spreading to the entire head. The prognosis for intertrochanteric osteotomy in such cases is uncertain; under certain conditions, the TPP might therefore be considered an alternative. As noted by Rüther et al. (see Chap. 9, this volume), in patients with femoral head necrosis, not only should radiographs, scanning and computed tomography (CT) be carried out, but also magnetic resonance imaging (MRI), because the necrosis might not necessarily be restricted to the femoral head only. Frequently, the femoral neck is also affected, at least partially, in which case implantation of a TPP might not be adequate. In such special cases of femoral neck necrosis, with an extension of the necrosis into the femoral neck area, implantation of a standard intramedullarly anchored prosthesis would be more appropriate.

Following healing of peri- and sub-trochanteric fractures, obliteration of the femoral medullary cavity as a result of osseous scars and incorrect fixation occasionally takes place, with the result that intramedullary fixation of a prosthesis is not possible. The TPP is an alternative solution in such cases. The same applies for unsatisfactory results following intertrochanteric osteotomy. The TPP has proved to be suitable for rare hip conditions such as dense osteoma or osteopetrosis.

In traumatic affections, as in fractures of the femoral neck, the TPP should only be implanted if the base of the femoral neck is intact (axial radiograph).

Contra-indications

Contra-indications are based on significant disturbances of the anatomy, of the relationship of axes and the trophic activity of the bone. The general contra-indications for total hip endoprostheses also apply for the TPP.

Implantation of a TPP is contra-indicated in patients with pronounced coxa vara, coxa valga and perhaps in those with a short, narrow femoral neck. As the acetabulum is also affected in these patients, endoprosthetic reconstructive corrective surgery using custom-made endoprostheses is usually required. The Girdlestone condition is a marginal indication. Metabolic disturbances of the bone, as well as severe osteoporosis with systemic disease, also belong to this marginal area. Conventional implants have proved effective in palliative surgery. Early relief from hip pain and patient mobilization are the principal objectives of treatment.

Surgical Technique

Preoperative Planning

For preoperative planning, a complete pelvic radiograph is needed, including a centralized one of the hip anteroposteriorly (AP) in neutral position (if possible with 20° medial rotation) and an axial radiograph. Radiographic templates are available for the planning of the positioning and selection of size of the TPP and for the selection of a suitable acetabular cup, respectively.

The most important associated criteria for the correct implantation of a TPP are as follows:

1. The TPP must be implanted with a physiological femoral shaft-neck angle of 125°–130° in order to allow the resultant hip-joint force to act physiologically, in magnitude and direction, on the femoral neck, thus giving rise to predominantly compressive forces.
2. The thrust plate must rest in full contact with the strongest part of the medial cortical bone of the femoral neck.

Only with correct positioning along the axis of the femoral neck can the TPP rest on a sufficiently thick portion of the medial cortical bone of the femoral neck.

The following basic values must be determined:

1. Angle of inclination (α) 125°–130° (femoral shaft-neck angle)
2. Distance between the tuberculum innominatum and the entry point of the central bolt (a)
3. Distance between the resection plane of the femoral neck and the trochanter minor (b).

After determining the size of the TPP using a template, these three basic values can be measured from the radiograph. The values α, a and b can be directly measured during the operation and compared with the preoperative plan (Fig. 3).

If it is attempted to place the TPP in a valgus position of more than 140°, there is a risk of the thrust plate no longer being seated on strong cortical bone. The lateral plate could then no longer fit onto the concave surface below the tuberculum innominatum. Being positioned too low, its upper part does not

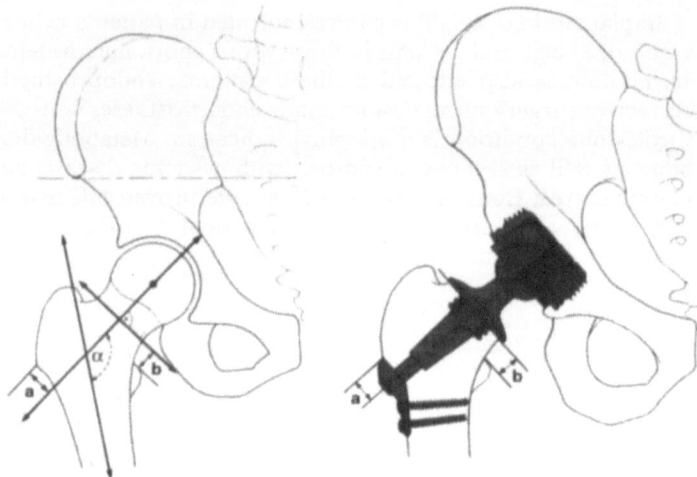

Fig. 3. Preoperative planning. The femoral neck angle of inclination (α) 125°–130°, the distance *a* from the tuberculum innominatum to the entry point of the central bolt and the distance *b* from the resected face of the femoral neck to the trochanter minor are measured

seat properly but projects from the straight portion of the femoral diaphysis. The head of the central bolt may also jam.

With the TPP in a valgus position, the difference in axial stiffness between bone and implant might cause oscillating movement of the central bolt in the lateral plate with each load cycle. Furthermore, in the presence of a valgus position of the TPP, the full cross-section of the femoral neck stump is subjected to compressive stresses and the medial cortical bone of the femoral neck is not sufficiently loaded. At the same time, the range of movement of the hip joint is restricted.

Considering deviations from the standard position, the valgus position is less serious than the varus position. Nevertheless, the TPP should not be implanted with a valgus femoral neck angle of more than 140°.

On the other hand, implantation of the TPP in a varus position is also unsuitable, because of high shear forces which encourage the thrust plate to slide transversely downwards. In an extreme varus position, the lower portion of the lateral plate with the two cortical screws might not rest against the lateral cortical bone of the femur. The TPP should therefore not be implanted with a varus femoral neck angle of less than 120° (Fig. 4).

Surgical Approach to the Hip Joint

The choice of approach is left to the surgeon, who may rely upon his personal surgical experiences. The anterior–lateral approach according to Watson-Jones, the transgluteal according to Bauer and the southern exposure of Moore are used most frequently. The Watson-Jones approach is not favourable for

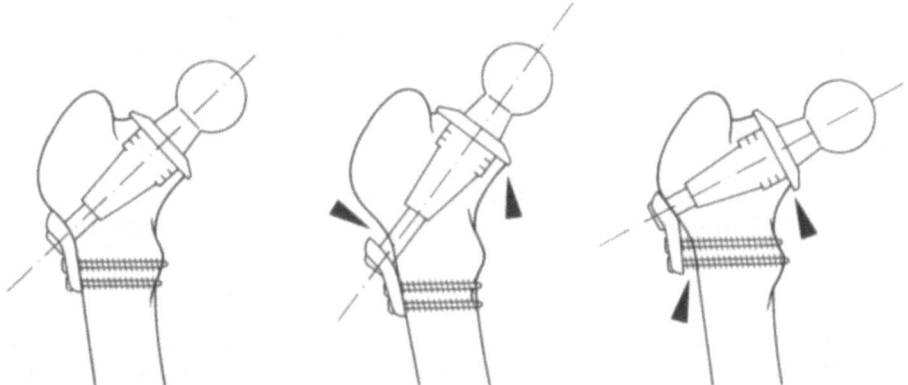

Fig. 4. The thrust plate prosthesis (TPP) must not be implanted at a femoral neck angle of more than 140° or less than 120° (see text). *Left*, 127° (normal); *middle*, 140° (valgus); *right*, 115° (varus). *Middle, right*, left-hand *arrowheads* show where the lash does not fit the contour of the femur; right-hand *arrowheads*, the bone is either exposed to relative stress relief in valgus (*middle*) or excessive shear forces in varus (*right*)

muscular individuals due to the restricted space in the area of the fossa trochanterica (despite partial dissection of the abductors) and the acetabulum. Occasionally, with this approach the tensor nerve might also be damaged. All these exposures leave the pelvitrochanteric muscles to a large extent unimpaired.

During exposure and surgical preparation of the femoral neck and the lateral femoral cortical bone, the periosteum is only removed to the extent necessary to ensure that no soft tissue is interposed between the thrust plate and the femoral neck stump and between the lateral plate and its underlying cortical bone. We prefer diathermic haemostasis for the smaller vessels. During the operation, when using the oscillating saw, the step drill and face-cutting reamer, regular rinsing with Ringer's solution is carried out with immediate suction removal.

Special Instruments

The TPP instrumentation contains standard drills, 4.5 mm and 3.2 mm for the cortical screws, with the corresponding 3.5-mm hexagon key, Kirschner wires, a pneumatic drill with angled drive and bayonet connector, and an oscillating saw.

There are some special instruments to facilitate implantation. The following are especially worthy of mention:

- *Drilling guide* (clamp, drilling bush, alignment guide) and centering disk with impactor.
- 10.5-mm *step drill*.

- *Tapered reamer.* This is used for preparing the bed for the mandrel of the prosthesis in the occasionally hardened cancellous bone of the femoral neck stump.
- *Face-cutting reamer.* This has a guide rod and a sleeve for tissue protection. Its purpose is to ream the surface of the resected femoral neck flat and down to the pre-determined length.
- A No. 6 *hexagon key* with a handle is provided for the central bolt.
- The TPP with its guide pin is seated in place with a special *impactor*.

Surgical Technique

Apart from the generally accepted rules for any surgical procedure, the surgeon should have a clear understanding of this new system concept before implanting the TPP.

The biological tolerance to errors of implantation of femoral stem prostheses with respect to size, position or relationship to the anatomical axes, as well as the method of fixation, is often amazing. The biological tolerance of the TPP to implantation errors is, however, lower.

The surgical technique involves no special difficulties. As noted above, the TPP is implanted along the longitudinal axis of the femoral neck at a physiological shaft angle of 125°–130°. After exposure of the hip joint and preparation of the centring hole in the lateral femoral cortical bone below the tuberculum innominatum, the femoral head is resected at the top of the neck. Following lateral rotation of the leg, the target plate is fitted on the stump of the femoral neck. The drilling guide is then mounted and fitted into the centring hole in the lateral–proximal femoral cortex. The central guide hole is then drilled from the lateral side in order to machine the femoral neck stump with the designated face-cutting reamer. Before the TPP is implanted, we recommend the implantation of a cementless acetabular cup (e.g. the cementless Balgrist cup). Following fixation of the thrust plate in the femoral neck, the central bolt of correct length is screwed in through the lateral plate, which is fastened with two cortical bone screws (Figs. 5–10).

In order to prepare the entry point of the central bolt, i.e. the area under the tuberculum innominatum within which the lateral plate will be placed, we recommend a minimum dissection of the vastus lateralis muscle. We leave a strip of muscle fascia about 1 cm wide attached to the insertion area at the tuberculum innominatum for easier reattachment of the muscle later. The area for the lateral plate must be cleared of soft tissue and periosteum. The entry point (centring hole for the step drill) marked with the 4.5-mm drill should be on the lateral side in the middle of the femoral shaft. The distance *a* is measured. Any irregular osteophytes possibly overlapping the femoral neck stump must be removed using bone forceps so that the cortical bone is visible all around. The centring disk can then be placed in the middle of the femoral neck stump without difficulty (Fig. 11).

The face-cutting reamer with the tissue protector is mounted in the angled drive (bayonet connection). The guide rod inserted through the femoral neck stump prevents the face-cutting reamer from tilting.

Fig. 5. Drilling guide in position

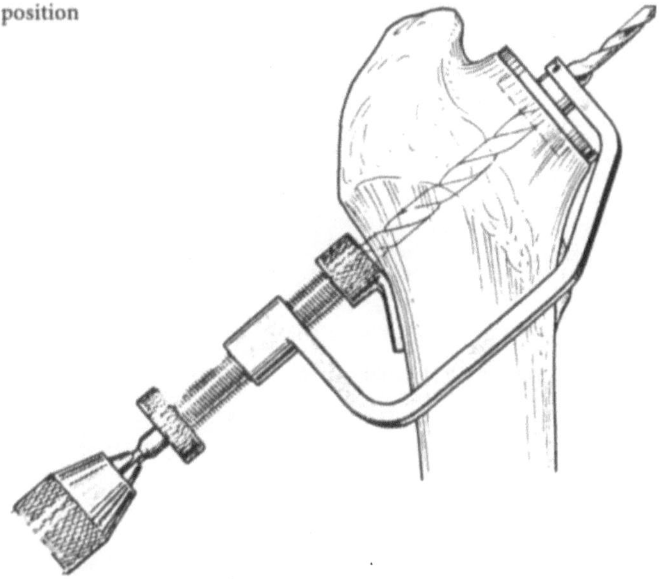

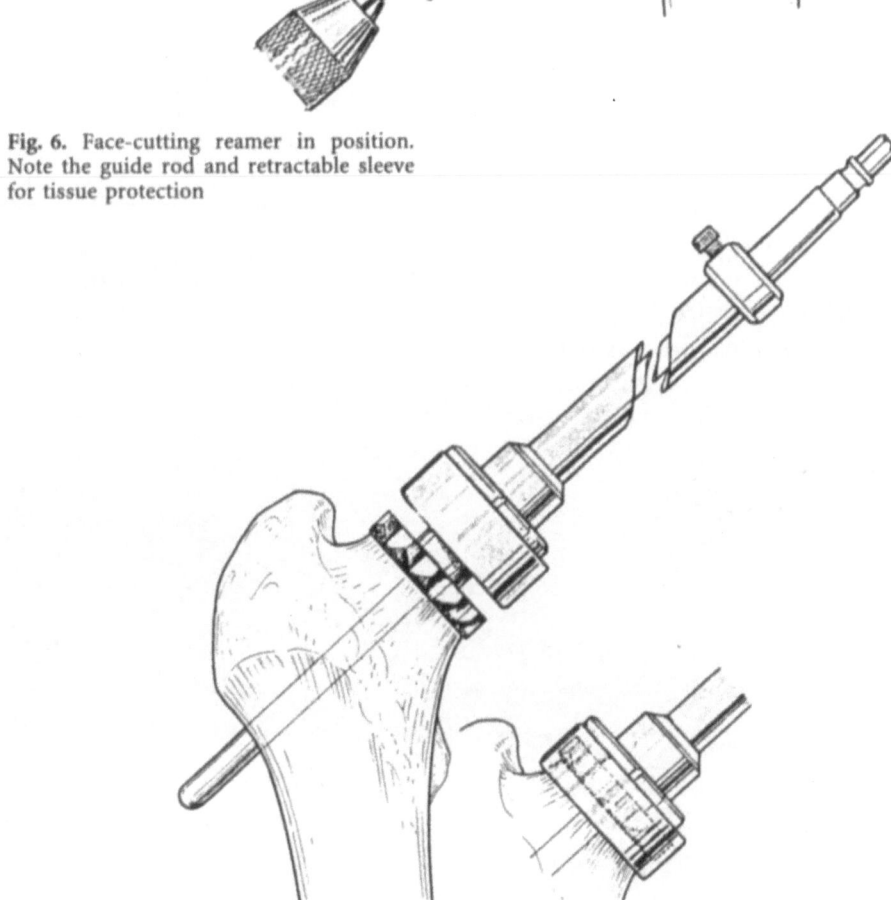

Fig. 6. Face-cutting reamer in position. Note the guide rod and retractable sleeve for tissue protection

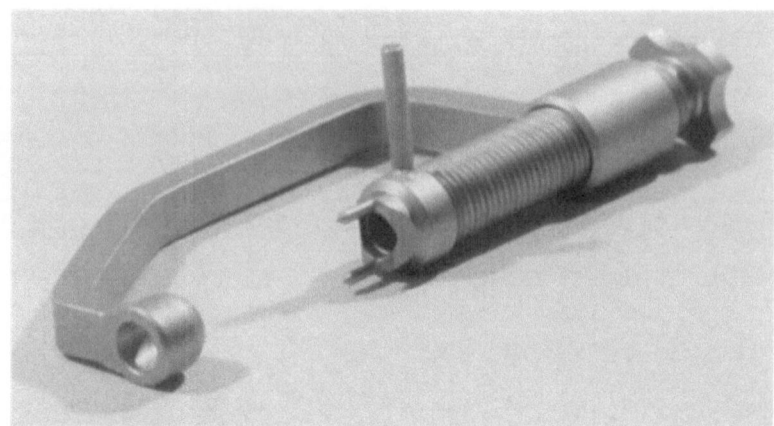

Fig. 7. Current type of drilling guide

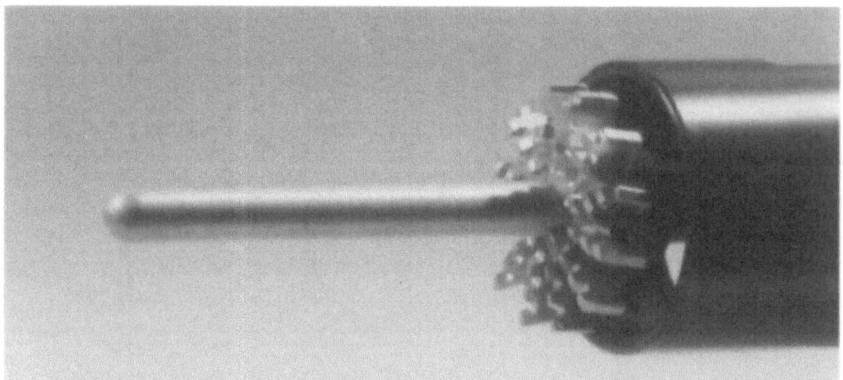

Fig. 8. Face-cutting reamer seen from below

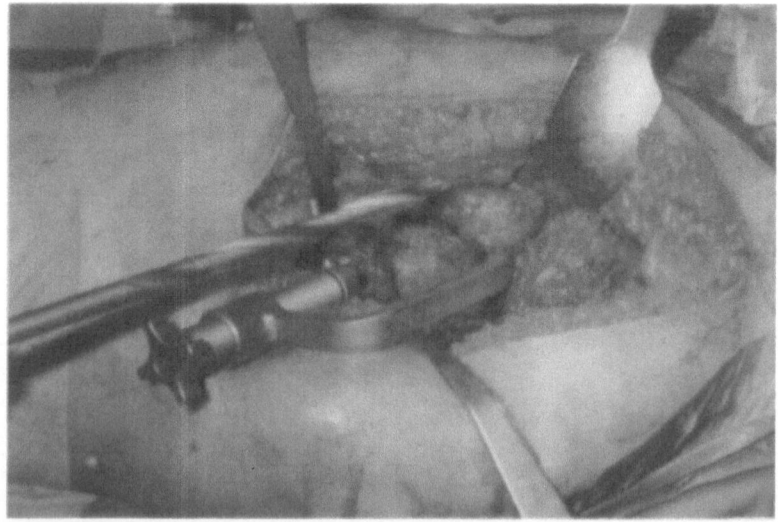

Fig. 9. Corresponding peri-operative view of the drilling guide in position

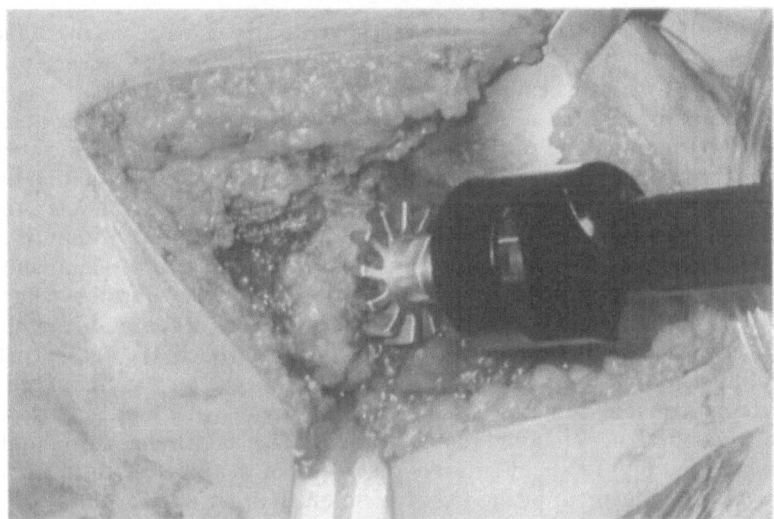

Fig. 10. Corresponding operation site of the face-cutting reamer

Insertion of the guide rod into the femoral neck stump may be difficult until the surgeon becomes acquainted with the orientation. Since the face of the femoral neck stump must be reamed in the pre-determined plane, correct insertion of the guide rod is essential. If the direction of the guide hole cannot be determined, it is useful to temporarily insert a Steinmann pin to visualize the direction. Sometimes the ilio-tibial tract running over the entrance of the guide hole on the lateral aspect of the femur prevents the guide rod from emerging. If necessary, the tractus may be split at the appropriate location.

Fig. 11. Due to asymmetrically protruding osteo-phytes, the centre of the femoral neck stump cannot always be determined. c, true centre of the femoral stump; c', false centre of the femoral stump due to the presence of an osteophyte

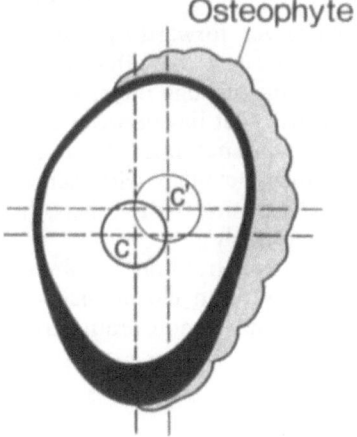

In the area of the medial cortical bone, the surface of the femoral neck stump must be flat and intact. The distance b to the lesser trochanter is measured using a flexible ruler or an opened Kocher clamp.

The exposure of the acetabulum, which is associated with the pushing aside of the proximal end of the femur, is left to the discretion of the surgeon.

The femur is externally rotated (if necessary with flexion) so that the femoral neck stump can be pushed away from the pelvis using a Hohmann retractor. It is also possible to internally rotate the femur (if necessary with flexion) so that the femoral neck stump can be pushed to the rear using a Hohmann retractor placed on the dorsal rim of the acetabulum. Care must be taken that the Hohmann retractors do not damage the periphery of the surface of the femoral neck stump. When using the Watson-Jones approach, the dorsal cortical bone of the femoral stump may occasionally be damaged on account of the restricted room available, but this is insignificant provided the medial cortical bone of the femoral neck stump remains intact. The acetabular cup should be implanted with only slight anteversion, or rather in a neutral position, in order to avoid impingement of the thrust plate on the rear edge of the cup in extreme joint positions (maximum extension and external rotation). Following implantation, the cup is protected with a gauze swab.

The correct size of thrust plate may be selected using the corresponding trial disk. It is necessary to remove hard cancellous bone from the femoral neck stump using small hollow chisels so that the "pedicles" under the thrust plate have sufficient space to avoid splitting the femoral neck stump. In addition, the bed for the thrust plate mandrel in the cancellous bone is prepared, if required, by using the tapered reamer, which is inserted up to two thirds of its length. Normally, the TPP is inserted by using an impactor, compressing the cancellous bone.

Insertion of the implant is always done with the guide pin screwed in, which has markings to determine the proper length of the central bolt. The thrust plate must lie flat on the strongest cortical bone of the femoral neck. Following removal of the guide pin, the central bolt is inserted through the lateral plate into the thrust plate and tightened. The central bolt may sometimes not properly engage with the thread of the thrust plate. The central bolt may then be driven forward by using one or two gentle hammer blows.

The correct length of the central bolt is checked by using the depth gauge in the hole through the proximal tapered end of the TPP. The correct length of the central bolt lies between the two marks on the depth gauge.

If, for anatomical reasons, there is a gap at the upper part of the lateral plate, it may be filled with cancellous bone. The lateral plate should be placed carefully under the tuberculum innominatum so as to allow the fascia lata to move freely.

The central bolt is tightened firmly once more before inserting the locking wire. Wound closure is performed and intra-articular, subfascial and subcutaneous Redon drains are inserted.

Postoperative Care

The postoperative care of patients with a freshly implanted TPP is in accordance with standardized guidelines commonly used in almost all clinics for conventional implants.

The postoperative stabilization of the leg is accomplished with an antirotation foam splint. The Redon drains are removed after 48 h. Early mobilization for reasons of thrombo-embolic prevention is an undisputed necessity. The patient is only discharged after sound healing of the wound is assured. Full weight-bearing should not begin for 6 weeks.

In the radiological follow-up examinations, it is important to assess the contact surface between the femoral neck stump and the thrust plate. For the AP and the optional axial X-rays, the hip joint must be centred with appropriate medial rotation, which can be checked using an image intensifier (see "Clinical Results").

Peri-operative Complications

In general, complications occur because the individual steps of the operation are not executed as prescribed:

1. The anteversion of the femoral neck must be considered when drilling the guide hole from the lateral side. When the longitudinal axis of the foot on the operating table is vertical, the axis of the femoral neck is horizontal (which can be verified, if needed, by feeling the ventral surface of the femoral neck with the forefinger). The centring hole below the tuberculum innominatum on the lateral side (halfway between the ventral and dorsal circumference of the cortex) must be checked with the finger. Central drilling of the femoral neck with the step drill ensures that the thrust plate can be implanted centrally without weakening of the cortical bone of the femoral neck or, worse, perforating it.
2. If the target plate (and thus the drilling guide) is mounted eccentrically on the femoral neck stump (because, for example, remaining osteophytes obstruct the view of the centre of the femoral neck stump), there is a risk of an eccentric hole, with the possible complication of perforating the dorsal femoral neck (see above). In such a case, the central hole should be started again in the correct position, and any defects should be filled with cancellous bone (femoral head).
3. During face reaming of the femoral neck stump or when the femoral neck stump is pushed away from the pelvis with a Hohmann retractor during implantation of the acetabular cup, small pieces of the cortical wall of the femoral neck stump may be broken off. No special action is needed in such a case, provided the thrust plate sits firmly on the medial cortical bone of the femoral neck stump. In other cases, filling with cancellous bone (femoral head) may be considered.
4. The "pedicles" of the thrust plate may press on the inside of the cortical bone of the femoral neck and cause it to split. Consequently, attention must

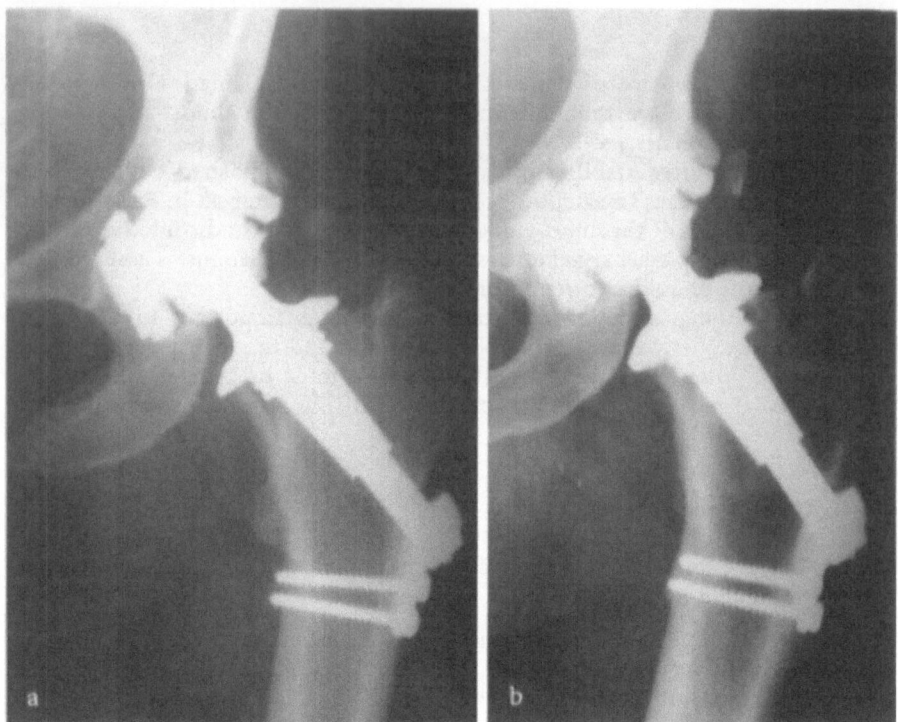

Fig. 12a,b. The fracture of the femoral neck stump during the operation consolidates with delayed postoperative weight-bearing. The thrust plate prosthesis (TPP) has been combined with a cementless Balgrist socket. (Courtesy of Dr. U. Schwarzenbach)

be paid to ensure that there is adequate space by using hollow chisels before implanting the TPP. Fractures due to bursting of the narrow femoral neck stump rarely occur at this stage of the operation. Although such a fracture, given otherwise stable implantation conditions, will heal without difficulties by longer reduced weight-bearing of the hip postoperatively, this complication should be avoided (Fig. 12).

Clinical Results

The field study performed in conjunction with the Balgrist University Clinic in Zurich was a valuable experience. It gave us the opportunity to present our unconventional hip implant to the orthopaedic community and to promote a critical exchange of ideas.

The field study permitted a numerically wider trial of the TPP. Furthermore, it provided specialist colleagues who had not been involved in the development and manufacture of the TPP, or in its initial clinical use, a chance to evaluate the implant without prejudice.

The first clinical experiences gained with the help of unbiased surgeons enabled us to set reasonable limits with regard to indications and further optimization of the surgical technique.

In the first series, there were 16 failures among a total number of 64 TPP implantations. These failures were caused by technical errors during the operation ($n=4$), material fatigue fractures in the lateral plate ($n=6$), infection ($n=4$) and others of unknown cause ($n=2$). The high failure rate at the beginning was partly due to technical and material complications, and partly due to inadequate implantations, either through inexperienced surgical technique or through the inadequate consideration of indications. Subsequently, the second series from 1988 and third series from 1992 have had no such complications to date.

The main indications are primary coxarthrosis (63%) and femoral head necrosis (16%); other indications being post-traumatic coxarthrosis (9%) and conditions following congenital hip dysplasia (6%). Coxarthrosis following slipped epiphyses and Perthes' disease, rheumatic coxitis and unsatisfactory intertrochanteric osteotomies are rarer. During the study, the mean patient age was 53.2 years (range, 19.9–78 years), with 74 men and 31 women. The average Harris hip score was 83 points. The survival curves (Kaplan-Meier) for the joint field study in Chur and Zurich are very similar (78% after 10 years, $n=166$).

Attention is drawn to the fact that in all of the revision operations carried out in the Canton's Hospital in Chur which were necessary after 10 years due to polyethylene cup wear, another TPP or a cementless stem prosthesis was able to be implanted (eight of 115). In the beginning, polyethylene cups were used in all TPP implantations. Despite good results on the femoral side, complications from the polyethylene falsely lowered the statistics for the TPP.

Compared with the first prosthesis model, significant improvements have been achieved in the second and third TPP series with regard to manufacturing, design and the material of the lateral plate. Titanium alloys were used for the lateral plate as well as for the thrust plate.

The danger of embolism through cement, fatty tissue, etc., which can occur as a result of drilled holes and pressure increases in the intramedullary space, is not relevant to the TPP.

The TPP is also different from prostheses with intramedullary fixation with respect to rotational stability, since the question is not applicable.

Fig. 13. Due to antetorsion of the femoral neck, the lateral plate sits behind and below the trochanter major

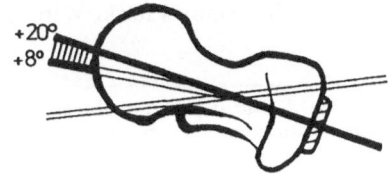

+20°
+8°

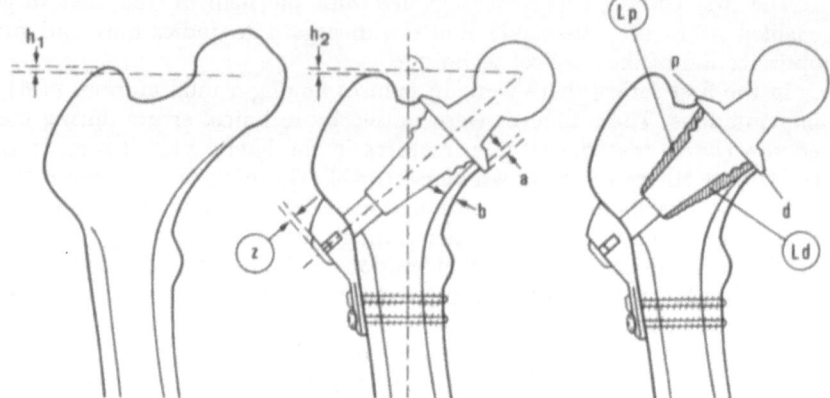

Fig. 14. Change in vertical position of joint centre to greater trochanter (h_1, h_2), tilt (a), thickness of medial cortical bone (b), radiolucent zones along the disk component (Lp, Ld) and subsidence of the central bolt (z). (Courtesy of Dr. R. Hauser)

Radiological Assessment

Radiological follow-up examinations which provide information as to the status of the TPP fixation, are analysed using "regions of interest" according to Hauser (see Chapter 5, this volume):

As with conventional prostheses with intramedullary fixation, six regions of interest according to Hauser may be identified for the TPP (Fig. 14). Of primary interest is the medial and lateral osseous contact surface between the thrust plate and the femoral neck stump. A specific radiograph is necessary (centred on the femoral neck with 20° medial rotation of the leg), so that the bone of the femoral neck stump under the thrust plate may be seen. The full cortical and cancellous bone structure of the proximal end of the femur is compared with the standard and/or preoperative condition. If necessary, the image converter is used to centre the hip joint. When appropriate, a check is also made of possible movement of the threaded bolt through the lateral plate as a result of loosening or resorption in the femoral neck stump. If there are no other clinical and radiological problems, the loosened threaded bolt can be tightened in ambulatory surgery.

Postoperatively, the thrust plate should sit directly on the medial cortical bone of the femoral neck. With a TPP implanted at the physiological femoral

Fig. 15a–d. Thrust plate prostheses (TPP) implanted at **a** a physiological femoral neck angle and **b** in an extreme valgus position. **c,d** Radiological follow-up examinations confirm the two types of loading of the femoral neck stump. The TPP implanted at a physiological femoral neck angle shows bone structure under the thrust plate scarcely deviating from the physiological pattern, whereas with the valgus position, atrophy of the medial cortical bone of the femoral neck and at the same time a thickening of the cancellous structures in the upper lateral portion of the femoral neck stump can be seen. (Fig. 15d courtesy of Dr. G. Gruber)

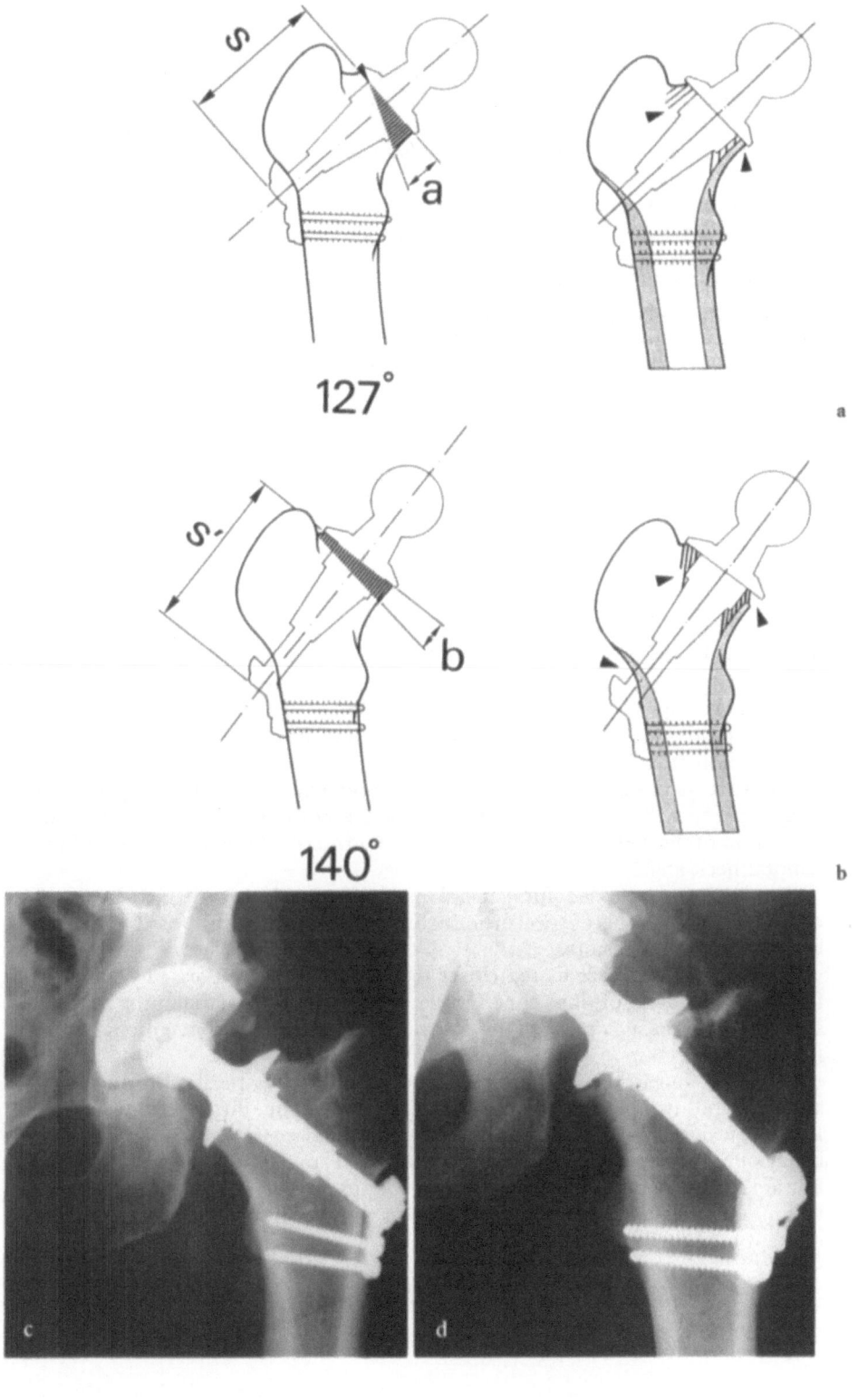

127°

140°

neck angle, the medial cortical bone of the femoral neck is retained. Additionally, after an average of 4–6 months, denser cancellous bone forms around the medial "pedicle", creating direct support through strong bundles of cancellous bone.

On the other hand, with the TPP implanted in the valgus position, these medial bundles of cancellous bone become voluminous to the detriment of the medial cortical bone of the femoral neck and are then the only supporting elements available. The medial cortical bone of the femoral neck is frequently atrophied and slightly rounded. In contrast to the physiological condition, the upper and outer area of the femoral neck with a valgus position is subject to compressive forces, so that functional densification of the cancellous bone can be seen on the radiograph. When implanted within the range of angular tolerance (femoral shaft-neck angle), the TPP is stable. If a TPP is implanted in a varus position, the mechanical situation is clearly less favourable than in an extreme valgus position, especially with respect to functional bone remodelling (Fig. 15).

Conclusions

The particular significance of the TPP as an alternative method of treatment to the classical cemented or cementless femoral prosthesis with intramedullary fixation is the restoration of equilibrium in load transfer between implant and bone, which approaches physiological conditions.

The long-term use attained with the TPP to date has demonstrated the range of indications that should be considered.

The successful outcome of hip-joint replacement using a TPP depends on careful preoperative planning and execution according to simple rules. Implantation of the TPP must be made within a prescribed tolerance range of the femoral neck angle of 120°–140°.

The TPP was released for general use only after more than 15 years of clinical experience because a meaningful evaluation is only possible on the basis of long-term results.

With the TPP, we are a step closer to the concept of a more physiological functional loading of the bone, while simultaneously maintaining a conservative approach compared to the relatively invasive, conventional stem fixation.

Bone reaction to the TPP after over 10 years in vivo, results in solid bony support and trouble-free trophic activity under the thrust plate surface. Radiological follow-up examinations and scans demonstrate this adaptive bone behaviour. In particular, the histology of a TPP retrieved post-mortem after 8 years in vivo confirms optimal bone adaptation to the TPP (see Chap. 3, this volume). Bone adaptation and good clinical results validate the biomechanical concept of the TPP.

References

1. Ballard WT, Callaghan J, Sullivan P, Johnston R (1994) The result of improved cementing techniques for total hip arthroplasty in patients less than fifty years old. J Bone Joint Surg 76A: 959–964
2. Bonola A (1953) La résection-reconstruction de la hanche par prothèse acrylique à amarrage sous-trochanterien. Rev Chir Orthop 39: 667–669
3. Dorr LD, Luckett M, Conaty JP (1990) Total hip arthroplasties younger than 45 years. A 9 10 year follow up study. Clin Orthop 260: 215–219
4. Freeman MAR (1978) Total surface replacement hip arthroplasty. Clin Orthop 134: 2–7
5. Freeman MAR, Cameron HU, Brown GC (1978) Cemented double cup arthroplasty of the hip. Clin Orthop 134: 45–52
6. Gambier R, Ricciardi L (1955) Tentative di artroplastica dell'anca con trapianto metallico totale di articolazione. Atti SIOT 40: 92
7. Huggler AH, Jacob HAC (1984) The uncemented thrust plate prosthesis. In: Morscher E (ed) The cementless fixation of hip endoprostheses. Springer, Berlin Heidelberg New York, pp 125–129
8. Huggler AH, Jacob HAC, Bereiter H, Haferkorn M, Ryf C, Schenk R (1993) Long-Term results with the uncemented Thrust Plate Prosthesis (TPP). Acta Orthop Belg 59 [Suppl I]:215–223
9. Huiskes R (1979) Some fundamental aspects of human joint replacement. Dissertation, Technische Hogeschool Eindhoven
10. Jackson Burrows H (1971) Replacement of tumours affecting bone by major internal prostheses. Biomedical engineering and its clinical application in orthpaedic surgery. British Council, London
11. Jacob HAC, Huggler AH (1978) Experimentelle Spannungsanalysen im menschlichen Oberschenkelknochen-Modell mit und ohne Prothese. Forschungsheft, Technische Rundschau, Sulzer, pp 73–83
12. Jacob HAC, Huggler AH (1980) An investigation into biomechanical causes of prosthesis stem loosening within the proximal end of the human femur. J Biomech 13: 159–173
13. Jacob HAC, Huggler AH, Dietschi C, Schreiber A (1976) The mechanical function of subchondral bone as experimentally determined on the acetabulum of the human pelvis. J Biomech 9: 625–627
14. Judet J, Judet R (1950) The use of an artificial femoral head arthroplasty of the hip joint. J Bone Joint Surg 32B: 166–173
15. Judet R, Siguier M, Brumpt B, Judet T (1978) A non cemented total hip prosthesis. Clin Orthop 137: 74–84
16. Lord G, Marotte JH, Blanchard JP (1988) Arthroplasties totales de hanche madréporiques. A propos de 2688 cas. Rev Chir Orthop 74: 3–14
17. McKee GK (1966/67) Developments in total hip joint replacement. Symposium on lubrication and wear in living and artificial human joints, vol 181, part 3J. Institution of Mechanical Engineers, London
18. McKee GK (1970) Development of total prothetic replacement of the hip. Clin Orthop 72: 85–103
19. Movin R (1955) Acrylic arthroplasty of the hip. J Bone Joint Surg 37B: 356–360
20. Mulroy RD, Harris W (1990) The effect of improved cementing techniques on component loosening in total hip replacement. J Bone Joint Surg 72B: 757–760
21. Perren SM, Huggler AH, Russenberger M, Allgöwer M, Mathys R, Schenk R, Willenegger H, Müller ME (1969) The reaction of cortical bone to compression. Acta Orthop Scand [Suppl] 125: 19
22. Picchio AA (1960) La ricostruzione dell'articolazione coxo-femorale con endoprotesi articolata nella l.c.a inventerata artrosica bilaterale. Atti SIOT Ed Pozzi, Roma, pp 541–559
23. Scholten R (1975) Über die Berechnung der mechanischen Beanspruchung in Knochenstrukturen mittels für den Flugzeugbau entwickeltes Rechenverfahren. Med Orthop Tech 6: 130–138
24. Schreiber A, Jacob HAC (1984) Loosening of the femoral component of the ICLH double cup hip prothesis. Acta Orthop Scand 55 [Suppl 207]: 1–34

25. Schreiber A, Jacob HAC, Suezawa Y, Huggler AH (1984) First results with the Thrust Plate Total Hip Prothesis. In: Morscher E (ed) The cementless fixation of hip endoprotheses. Springer, Berlin Heidelberg New York, pp 130–132
26. Trentani C, Vaccarino F (1978) The Paltrinieri-Trentani hip joint resurface arthroplasty. Clin Orthop 134: 36–40
27. Wagner H (1978) Surface replacement arthroplasty of the hip. Clin Orthop 134: 102–130
28. Wiles P (1957/58) The surgery of osteoarthritic hip. Br J Surg 45: 488–497
29. Willert HG, Semlitsch M (1972) Histopathology associated with polymers and metals in total hip replacement. Gordon conference on science and technology of biomaterials, Tilton, USA, Aug 1972
30. Wolff J (1892) Das Gesetz über die Transformation der Knochen. Hirschwald, Berlin
31. Wroblewski BM (1993) Charnley low-friction arthroplasty of the hip. Long-term results. Clin Orthop 292: 191–201
32. Zanoli R (1956) Les prothèses acryliques dans la chirurgie de la hanche. Rev Chir Orthop 42: 330–331

CHAPTER 2

Biomechanical Principles and Design Details of the Thrust Plate Prosthesis

H.A.C. Jacob

Introduction

As is probably the case for all substantially successful innovations, the remarkably unique design of the thrust plate prosthesis (TPP) was not born of a sudden whim or a capricious desire to merely produce a hip joint replacement that radically differed from all other commonly known types, but emerged from an elaborate biomechanical investigation on the loosening of conventional, intramedullarly anchored hip prosthesis shafts. Therefore, to appreciate the principles on which the TPP is based, it is necessary to first review some of the earlier work done on this matter before proceeding to the TPP itself. This article therefore begins with a description of the experimental stress analysis that was carried out in the middle of the 1970s on models of the human pelvis and femur. The observations made during these early studies and the conclusions drawn from them virtually forced Arnold Huggler and myself to seek for a practicable solution that would overcome some of the biomechanical weaknesses of conventional prostheses. While considering all possible means of attaching a ball head to the proximal femur and bearing in mind that a successful prosthesis would be one that loads the bone in its immediate vicinity as physiologically as possible, we were suddenly captured by the simple idea of transmitting the hip joint force by means of a thrust plate, or washer, to the resected neck of the femur. From the birth of this idea, on 12 March 1976, up to the first implantation of a prototype in a 42-year-old man on 1 Februar 1978, various model investigations were carried out to test the mechanical behaviour of the prosthesis. This also involved reflections pertaining to the biocompatiblity of the materials chosen. Hence, the second part of this article deals with the basic design features of the TPP.

After the implantation of two prototypes in 1978, it was decided to introduce a first series of about 50 prostheses (it turned out to be 64) from 1981 onwards. This first small series called for design modifications of the prototypes to meet production and safety demands. Surgical handling experience and the advent of titanium and titanium alloys as a favourable implant material called for still further design improvements, which were then introduced in 1986. Finally, the encouraging clinical results obtained with the first series of TPP after an implantation period of more than 10 years prompted us to further improve the design; it now has less components than before, while allowing for more efficient manufacturing and assembly procedures.

During the whole period of design development, any modifications suggested by either orthopaedic surgeons, the manufacturer, or the distributor have been carefully reviewed, since complying with one desire might well introduce a problem elsewhere. This constantly called for compromises which, however, were not allowed to encroach on the biomechanical principles on which the TPP is based. Although the TPP was conceived over 15 years ago, its principal characteristics have thus remained unaltered up to today, as shown in the third part of this presentation.

Those sections of this chapter which relate to already published material have been kept as short as possible but hopefully still contain sufficient information to allow the reader to follow, without reference to the original articles.

Biomechanical Investigations on the Loosening of Hip Implants

The following is a short account of investigations that were begun in the early 1970s when attempting to determine the cause of loosening of hip implants other than that commonly attributed to the bone cement. Faced with reports of over 25% loosenings within 5 years of implantation and in a joint venture with the Department of Orthopaedic Surgery, Balgrist, University of Zurich [1, 2], we first decided to carry out experimental investigations in the hope of finding the stress pattern within the bone of the loaded hip altered to such an extent by the implant that the resorption of bone in the vicinity of the implant could then be explained by Wolff's law.

Composite full-scale epoxy models of the human pelvis were made in which both the cortical and cancellous bone were simulated, i.e. the relationship of their respective elastic properties were in the same proportion as that observed in fresh bone. This was necessary to ensure that the load-sharing between these materials of varying density (and stiffness) was similar to that which might be expected physiologically. Tri-axial strain gauge rosettes were applied to the model in the area of the acetabulum (lateral and medial aspects) and to the semi-lunate subchondral surface of the acetabulum. The model also allowed strain gauge rosettes to be embedded within the cancellous material just superior to the roof of the acetabulum. Furthermore, strain gauge rosettes were applied to the cortical material at the interface between cortical and cancellous substance. The action of the abductor muscles was simulated by numerous strings attached to the pelvis and greater trochanter, while the model was loaded in one-legged stance by a vertical force applied just anterior to the promontorium. For more details of this investigation, please refer to the literature already published [1, 2].

The results showed that the pelvic bone is a perfect example of a true sandwich structure in which the cover plates (cortex) are highly stressed in tension or compression, while the core remains in a relatively lower stressed condition serving mainly to prevent collapse of the principle load-bearing limbs. It was also shown that the subchondral bone within the acetabulum (semi-lunate face) transmits the main part of the load in the form of membrane stresses from the hip joint to the rim of the acetabulum and then onto the cortical shell of the ilium.

It was precisely when discussing the results of this investigation that our attention was closely drawn to the force-transmitting function of cortical bone – as opposed to that of the cancellous material, in spite of the fascinating trabecular trajectories exhibited by the latter. Arnold Huggler and I extended the conclusions drawn from this investigation to the proximal end of the human femur, which resulted in the concept of the TPP even before we had carried out any investigations on the femur itself. Nevertheless, since the principle of the TPP is probably more comprehensible in the light of our investigations on the biomechanical causes of prosthesis stem loosening within the proximal end of the human femur, a brief review of this work is first presented.

A conventional intramedullarly implanted femoral endoprosthesis is at its best only a compromise. The great strength required of the prosthesis necessitates the use of metallic alloys with an unfortunately high Young's modulus of 110–240 kN/mm^2, while cortical and cancellous bone exhibit values of less than 20 kN/mm^2 and 1.5 kN/mm^2, respectively. Problems due to lack of stiffness compatibility between the implant and the surrounding bone might therefore be expected. As Wolff [3] showed, the bone is able to adapt itself, by remodelling, to existing conditions of mechanical loading. This, together with the relatively low Young's modulus of the intermediate layer of bone cement of about 0.3 kN/mm^2, might lead to conditions of load distribution between the stem of the prosthesis and the surrounding bone that might be acceptable after all. On the other hand, initial bone remodelling might also lead to an unstable condition that would only worsen, leading to inevitable failure of the device. To investigate this matter further, we carried out experimental stress analysis on epoxy models of the femur that were made in a similar fashion to the one of the pelvis described above, i.e. both the cortical and cancellous bone were simulated so that the relationship of their respective elastic properties was in the same proportion as that observed in fresh bone. Even the prosthesis employed was made of an aluminium alloy that exhibited a Young's modulus with an appropriate relationship to that of the generally employed CoCr material. For more detailed information, please refer to the literature already published [4].

A full-scale model of only the upper third of the femur was made (Fig. 1). A rig that simulated the pelvis was attached to the greater trochanter by means of strings, the latter simulating the action of the pelvi-trochanteric abductor muscles in one-legged stance. The model was loaded by means of weights applied to the "pelvis" to simulate body weight. In addition to 11 tri-axial strain gauge rosettes that were embedded in the meridional cross-section in the frontal plane, 48 similar rosettes were also placed on the outside of the model, as shown in Fig. 2. To obtain a proper comparison between the stress conditions in bone, both with and without a prosthesis, only a single model was used. Initially, strain measurements were carried out on the loaded intact model (without a prosthesis). Following this, the femoral head was cut away and a prosthesis intramedullarly implanted in the same model.

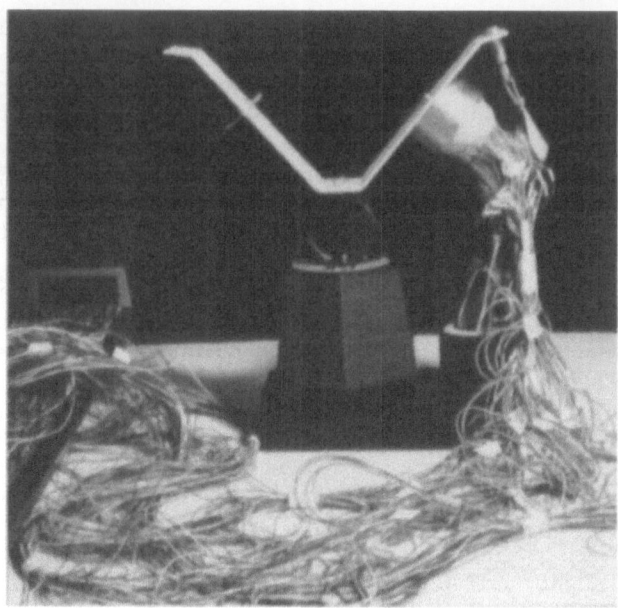

Fig. 1. The instrumented model, without prosthesis, loaded in one-legged stance

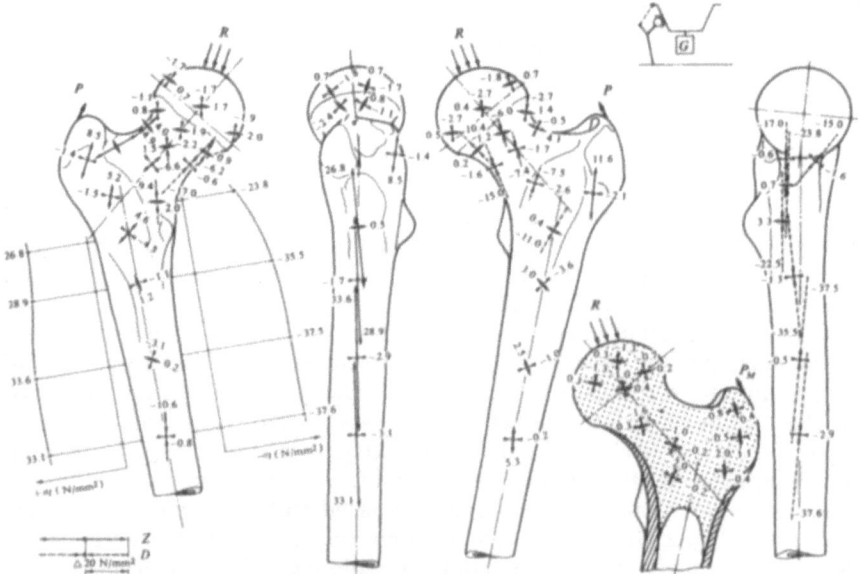

Fig. 2. Principal stresses in the physiological femur when standing on one leg, for a total body weight of 600 N. *Z*, tensile stresses (+); *D*, compressive stresses (-); *R*, hip joint force; *P*, muscle force

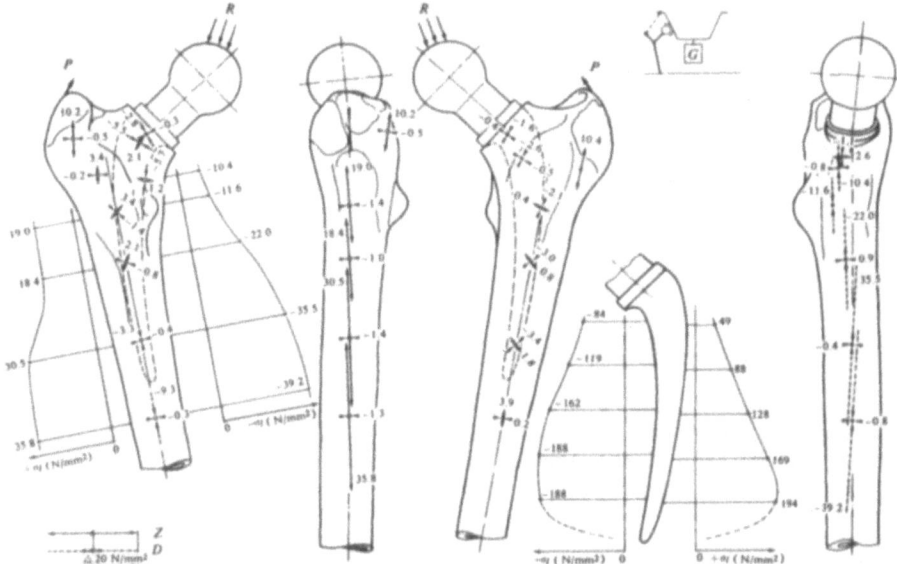

Fig. 3. Principal stresses in the femur with intramedullarly anchored prosthesis, for a total body weight of 600 N. *Z*, tensile stresses (+); *D*, compressive stresses (-); *R*, hip joint force; *P*, muscle force

A comparison of the results, in physiologically intact condition (Fig. 2) and after an intramedullarly anchored prosthesis was implanted (Fig. 3), clearly indicated the reduction of stress along the medial and lateral aspects of the femur with implant. At the proximal end, the reduction amounts to about 60% of the physiological stress. This reduction in stress, which probably gives rise to the commonly observed atrophy of bone in the region of the calcar in accordance with Wolff's law, is due to the high axial stiffness of the prosthesis stem compared with that of the surrounding bone [4].

Moreover, through resection of the femoral head, the continuity of bone is interrupted so that the bone in the immediate vicinity of the cut is no longer loaded by the forces that acted perpendicular to the area of cross-section (as physiologically occurs in the intact bone). Figure 4 illustrates the alteration of the stress pattern within the femoral neck on loading, before and after an intramedullarly anchored prosthesis has been implanted. It has long since been realized that the bone in the immediate vicinity of the plane of resection suffers inadequate loading, and several attempts have been made to rectify this by means of large neck collars and cobra-like flanges [5]. However, it has been shown [4, 5] that such contraptions have little or no effect, again because of the axial stiffness of the stem compared with that of the proximal femur; we therefore chose a different approach to this problem, as described below.

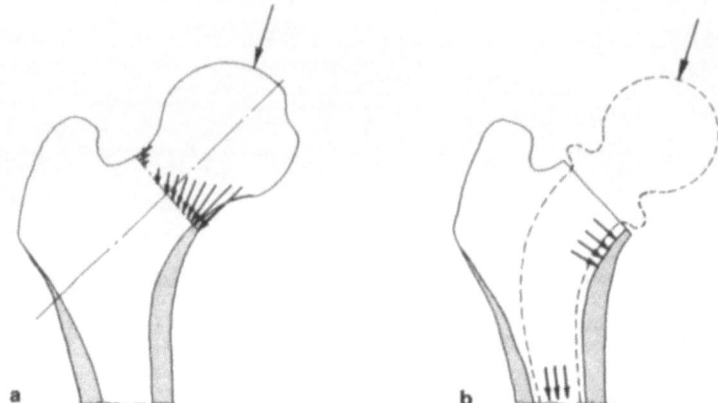

Fig. 4a,b. Difference in stress pattern (*arrows*) within the femoral neck. **a** Physiological state. **b** After implantation of an intramedullarly anchored prosthesis

Concept of the Thrust Plate Prosthesis and Preliminary Investigations

In the preceding section, the major biomechanical drawbacks of the conventional stem prosthesis were illustrated. It has been clearly shown that if a stem of necessarily strong material (and therefore usually of some high-strength metal, adequately dimensioned) is firmly attached to the surrounding bone such that no sliding motion can take place between bone and implant at any point along the interface, then the bone in the region of the proximal part of the femur will suffer stress relief and will cause bone resorption through mechanical inactivity. If, on the other hand, the stem is free to glide within the medullary canal and is furnished with a large collar that rests on the resected neck of the femur, the bone will be loaded as desired but relative motion between stem and surrounding bone will also certainly cause resorption of bone, probably leading to lateral migration of the prosthesis tip.

Considering the above, it becomes most evident that the stem must be eliminated from any future design. Simultaneously, the hip joint force must be transmitted by means of a flat plate to the neck of the femur and some contraption must be applied to prevent the flat plate from being lifted off the femoral neck. These are the essential features which had to be incorporated in a new prosthesis design.

Since the hip-joint force acts obliquely on the resected neck surface, there is not only a distinct tendency for a thrust plate to slip transversally, i.e. parallel to the plane of resection, but also for it to lift off at the cranio-lateral aspect of the neck. (Some tensile stresses might be present in this area of the physiological femur). To deal with this situation, we first envisaged an annular groove in the thrust plate which would contain the cortex of the femoral neck and thus prevent any transversal slipping motion relative to the bone. Tilting the thrust plate on the bone was to be prevented either by a slender rod passing along the

Fig. 5. The prototype thrust plate prosthesis (TPP) as implanted in two patients in 1978

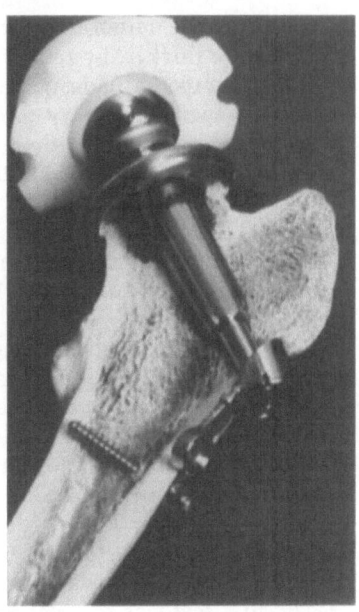

axis of the femoral neck down to the lateral cortex, which was maintained in a state of sufficient pre-tension, or by means of a rigid mandrel that also reached the lateral cortex just below the greater trochanter. The mandrel was required to deflect as little as possible under cantilever bending so as to ensure that the plane of the thrust plate would continue to remain unaltered as far as possible relative to the bone when loaded. Since the behaviour of bone under continuous static loading is unpredictable (it would probably remodel until the continuous static load has dropped to a very low value), it was decided to pursue only the rigid mandrel idea, as shown in Fig. 5.

Obviously, the thrust plate has to be seated on the femoral neck and attached to it in such a way that the former cannot slip transversally. This was accomplished by an annular recess in the plate which accomodated a short length (2 mm) of femoral neck. Any space left free within this annular groove was to be filled with bone cement so that the neck was virtually embedded in cement contained within the thrust plate.

The thrust plate was furnished with a central bore that allowed a mandrel to pass through until the latter was seated. From the lateral aspect, a central bolt was passed along the femoral neck axis to engage with a female thread within the mandrel, thus clamping the metaphysial bone between thrust plate and bolt head. A plate between the head of the bolt and the underlying lateral cortex permitted transmission and distribution of the bolt force to the bone. The central bolt, following the axis of the neck, passes through an area of the lateral cortex which is quite thin and is immediately below the greater trochanter. Since the thin layer of cortical bone cannot offer much resistance to transversal forces imposed by the bolt in a cranial direction, the lateral plate is also attached to the femoral cortex slightly distally, where the cortex becomes significantly thicker, by means of two cortical bone screws.

Following the basic design concept as mentioned above, the next step was to determine the preliminary dimensions of the various components as appropriately as possible and then carry out a rough theoretical estimate of the stresses involved. This was followed by a far more reliable stress analysis on full-scale epoxy models of the femur using materials for the prosthesis which would have the same stiffness relationship to the model femur as later on in the clinical setting. The components of the prosthesis were therefore made of the aluminium alloy Anticorodal-100 and were fitted to an epoxy femur as described above.

Nineteen tri-axial strain gauge rosettes of 3-mm grid length were applied to the proximal part of the femur, from 7 mm below the plane of neck resection up to just beyond the lateral plate in the region of the diaphysis. The prosthesis was so implanted that a femoral shaft-neck angle of 130° resulted. Strain measurements were carried out under the following conditions: (a) pre-tensioning of the central bolt alone, (b) one-legged stance with bolt tightened, and (c) one-legged stance with the bolt loosened. Loading of the model in one-legged stance was performed in a similar manner to that described above with intramedullarly anchored prostheses.

The first test was to determine the stress pattern in the bone on tightening the central bolt. The results showed that a tightening torque of 1.6 Nm (standard 8 mm thread, lightly oiled) gave rise to compressive stresses in the bone, 7 mm below the thrust plate, amounting to -6 N/mm^2 on the dorsal side and -4 N/mm^2 on the ventral surface.

The results obtained for one-legged stance, extrapolated and standardized for a body weight of 600 N, are shown in Fig. 6. No significant differences were observed between the stress pattern of the bone with the central bolt fully tightened or loose, and thus only this one diagram (Fig. 6) is shown here. This proved that, even if the central bolt has lost its pre-stress through bone remodelling, provided that the head of the central bolt is sufficiently guided to prevent oscillation in a cranio-caudal direction, the force transmission from prosthesis to bone remains the same.

Furthermore, a comparison of the stress pattern observed in a femur in its physiological state (Fig. 2) with that shown in Fig. 6 shows no significant differences, thus clearly indicating that the TTP is capable of loading the bone in a physiological manner.

The appropriate dimensions of the various components of the TPP then had to be determined and suitable materials chosen. Fortunately, we were able to make use of the broad spectrum of implantable materials available from Sulzer Bros. Ltd. [6] and decided to use CoCrMo alloys for the purpose, although manufacturing feasibility and lowest possible cost were major factors that had to be considered in the process.

Measurement of eight cadaver femora of patients between 22 and 81 years showed that the external neck diameter varied between 30 mm and 42 mm, with an average of 38 mm; the distance between the plane of neck resection and the intersection between neck axis and lateral cortex was between 49 mm

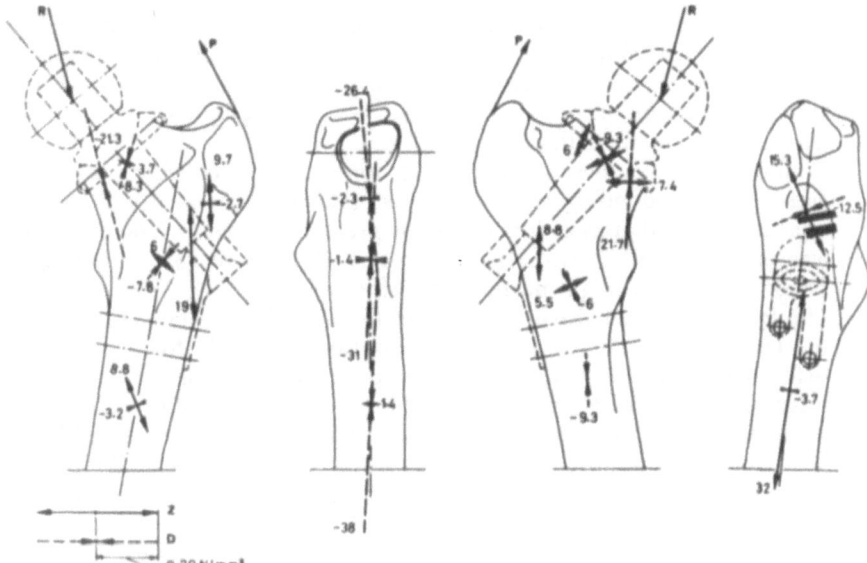

Fig. 6. Principal stresses in the femur with the thrust plate prosthesis (TPP) for a total body weight of 600 N. Z, tensile stresses (+); D, compressive stresses (-); R, hip joint force; P, muscle force

and 53 mm, with an average of 55 mm; and the femoral shaft-neck angle varied between 120° and 130°, with an average of 126°. Based on these principle dimensions, a total of four prototypes were made which exhibited the following main features:

- The *thrust plate* was circular and made of cast CoCrMo (Protasul -2). Two sizes were available, one with an outer diameter of 46 mm, and the other of 42 mm. The groove in one of the faces of the thrust plate for accommodation of the femoral neck was 3 mm deep with an outer diamter of 42 mm in the one size, and 38 mm in the other. The inner diameter of the groove was the same in both sizes, measuring 25 mm. A hole in the middle of the thrust plate allowed a mandrel of 16 mm in diameter to pass through and permitted seating of a spherical shoulder of the latter on the proximal face of the plate.
- The total length of the *mandrel* was 68 mm, and it was also made of cast CoCrMo. From one side of a spherical shoulder, it protruded about 45 mm into the femoral neck. Proximally, on the other side of the shoulder, it was furnished with a 16-mm-diameter cylindrical bearing surface that allowed a ball head with a corresponding blind hole to be slipped over it, thus forming a trunnion bearing. The distal part of the mandrel presented four ribs that locked into the surrounding cancellous bone, thus preventing rotation of the mandrel. A central bore within the mandrel accommodated a close-fitting bolt of 8 mm in diameter that fitted into a corresponding thread at the end of the bore.

- The *central bolt* of the prosthesis of 8-mm diameter was made of high-strength forged alloy CoNiCrMoTi (Protasul-10). Because of the danger of scoring and fretting between bolt and mandrel (adverse tribological properties of Protasul-10), it was decided to furnish the bolt with a plating of chromium, a method that was being practiced at that time [7]. The bolt exhibited a hemispherical head of 14 mm in diameter which was seated within a corresponding recess in a boss that was part of the lateral plate attached to the diaphysis just below the greater trochanter. The central bolt was manufactured in two lengths (93 and 83 mm) to cover the range of femoral sizes that might normally be expected.
- The *lateral plate* consisted primarily of the boss that contained the head of the central bolt and two straps that continued distally for about 35 mm before each was attached to the cortex by a cortical bone screw. The boss was made of Protasul-2, while the welded-on straps were of Protasul-10. The hemispherical head of the central bolt closely fitted into the bore within the boss so that, if and when the bolt head lifted off its seat, an axial movement of the bolt of up to about 2 mm within the bore was possible while still being radially guided. This ensured that even if the bolt became loose through bone remodelling, the TPP would continue to be constrained within the femur. A simple locking wire which passed through the head of the bolt and through slots in the boss prevented the bolt from turning loose if the pretension dropped off.
- *Ball heads* of 32 mm in diameter, made of cast CoCrMo, were available in three neck lengths in steps of 5 mm and could be fitted to the proximal end of the mandrel.

Before attempting to implant the prosthesis clinically, it was decided to carry out further laboratory testing. The first of these tests involved the loading of a TPP implanted in a fresh cadaver femur, and the second was to observe the behaviour of the prosthesis under repeated cyclic loading.

The fresh cadaver femur of about 20 cm in length was stripped of all muscle tissue with the exception of the abductor tendons, which were carefully preserved. The femur was held at its distal end in a tubular support of steel with its axis inclined 10° to the vertical (as in one-legged stance). The head was excised and the neck resected so that a plane normal to the neck axis with a femoral shaft-neck angle of 125° resulted. Resection was performed until the bone in the calcar area was of substantial thickness while leaving the neck to stand proud of the fossa trochanterica by about 4 mm. The neck was then prepared for receiving the mandrel after a central bore of 8 mm in diameter passing along the neck axis up to the lateral cortex had been made. The broad groove in the thrust plate was filled with bone cement, and while the cement was still in a soft state the thrust plate was pressed onto the femoral neck. The central bolt was introduced and tightened fully. After this, the two cortical bone screws were used to additionally fix the lateral plate to the cortex. A ball head with medium neck length (30 mm between centre of ball and resected neck) was fitted. A heavy jig that simulated the pelvis was furnished with an acetabular cup that fitted the ball head and was further connected to the femur by a gripping device that grasped the abductor tendons on the greater trochanter. The whole set-up was loaded in an Instron testing machine so that a force could be applied simulating body weight in one-legged stance.

While force was being applied, the position of the thrust plate on the femur was carefully observed so as to detect any transversal slipping or collapse of the underlying bone. The maximum force applied before the grip on the tendons gave way was about 1000 N (body weight). No relative movement or sign of disturbance was detected during the test. The same test was repeated with the central bolt loosened, i.e. with the bolt head just in contact with its seat. After the tendons had been regripped, a maximum force of about 1500 N (body weight) could be applied before they slipped again. Once again, no movement whatever was detected between the TPP and bone.

To test the endurance strength of the prosthesis, the TPP was assembled in a steel device that resembled the proximal femoral bone. Again, the thrust plate was rigidly fixed to the steel device with bone cement and the central bolt only lightly tightened to take up any slack. The device was held in a tilted position in an Amsler fatigue testing machine so that the prosthesis was loaded repeatedly in the physiological direction of hip joint force. The TPP was first subjected to 3.5×10^6 cycles between 200 N and 3200 N, then to 5×10^6 cycles between 300 N and 5300 N and finally to 5×10^6 cycles between 500 N and 8000 N. The test was carried out under ambient conditions at 2 c/s.

Following all these tests, which I conducted in 1977 at the Department of Stress Analysis and Material Behaviour in the General Research and Development Division of Sulzer Bros. Ltd., the TPP was implanted for the first time by Arnold Huggler in a 42-year-old hip patient in January 1978. This first implantation was followed by a second in the same year.

Fourteen months after implantation of the first TPP and 11 months after the 43-year-old patient had returned to work as a labourer, the central bolt broke, just at the level where the shaft emerged from the bore in the mandrel. The TPP was easily replaced by a conventional prosthesis, and the failed TPP components were sent for material investigation. The detailed metallurgical study of the retrieved components showed that crevice corrosion of the chromium plating on the bolt shaft had taken place, giving rise to a notch effect which, in the presence of high nominal stresses, led to fatigue failure of the bolt. This experience caused us to modify not only the dimensions of the bolt, but also to avoid the use of chromium plating in future by choosing another high-strength alloy with less tendency to fret and score.

In the meantime, the second TPP, which was similar to the first except that it had a shorter central bolt, continued to give excellent service (Fig. 7) until 5 years later, in 1983, a 73-year-old alpine farmer was unexpectedly lost through death.

After a watchful pause of 2 years, we continued with the implantation of the TPP, in a slightly modified version, from 1980 to 1985, during which period 64 implantations were carried out. The next section deals with details of all modifications and tests carried out from 1980 up to now.

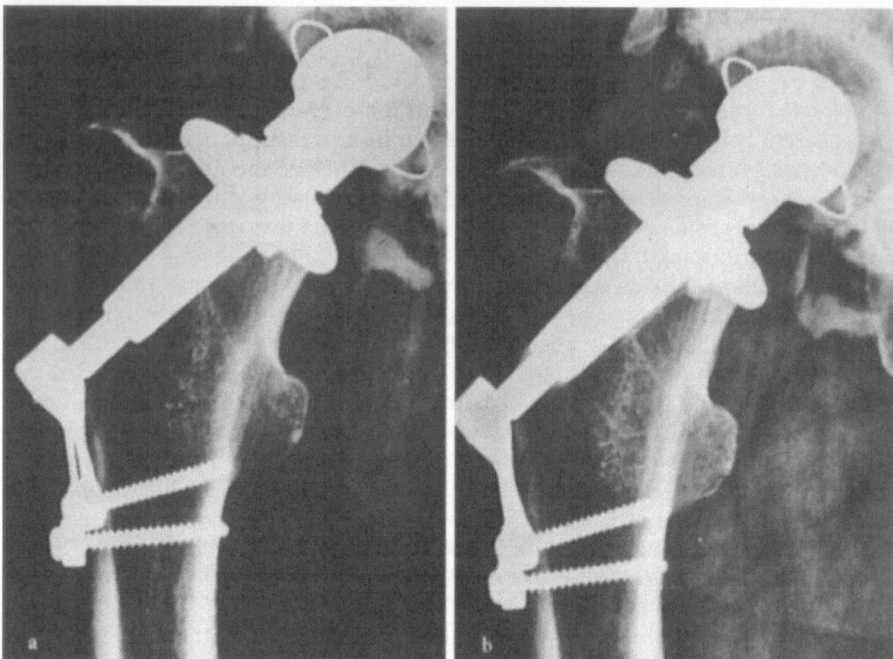

Fig. 7a,b. Male patient born in 1912. **a** Three months after implantation of a thrust plate prothesis (TPP) (September 1978). **b** Four years later (1982)

Design Details and Modifications from 1980 Onwards

First Series (1980–1987)

Following the successful implantation of the first two prototypes as mentioned above, it was decided to implant a small series of prostheses in two orthopaedic centres, in the Canton's Hospital, Chur, and in the University Hospital Balgrist, Zurich. This TPP series will be referred to as the first series.

It had since been definitely decided to avoid the use of bone cement completely; the surface of the thrust plate in juxtaposition with the bone was therefore given a rough structure to afford sufficient grip in resisting transversal slip. The best surface profile under the manufacturing conditions that had to be met with (low cost with hardly any interest on the part of the manufacturer at that time to envisage production of a series larger than about 50 prostheses) was to drill several closely set holes of 3 mm in diameter and 0.5 mm in depth, into the surface. This was to afford initial grip immediately after implantation and to encourage bone ingrowth later on. The surface was additionally roughened by shot-blasting. The inner and outer boundaries of the thrust surface were marked by rims that stood proud of the surface by 4 mm, thus forming a broad shallow groove between them to contain the resected neck of the femur. An additional protrusion extended past the 4-mm-high

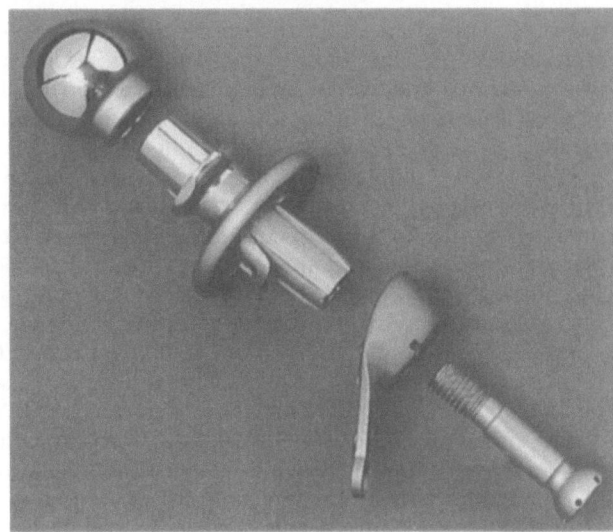

Fig. 8. The thrust plate prosthesis (TPP) of the first series (1980–1987)

inner rim by another 5 mm only on the caudal aspect so as to be able to rest against the inner surface of the calcar, should the thrust plate lose its grip on the underlying bone and slip downwards. This was only a security measure. The thrust plate, available in two sizes of 43- and 47-mm outer diameter, was rotationally symmetrical (Fig. 8) and made of cast CoCrMo alloy. The proximal end of the central hole that accommodated the mandrel opened into a 45° seat which fitted into the spherical shoulder on the mandrel.

The *mandrel* was also made of cast CoCrMo alloy and retained many of the principle dimensions of the prototypes. One main difference consisted in providing for a larger central bolt (10 mm in diameter instead of 8 mm). As in the prototypes, a shoulder with a spherical surface transmitted the hip-joint force to the thrust plate. The mandrel was available in two lengths to cover the requirements for all sizes of femora generally encountered; there were also two lengths of central bolt, so that altogether four combinations of sizes were available. (Later on in this first series of TPP, only the shorter mandrel was used in conjunction with one of four lengths of central bolt). The reason for this variety of sizes of bolts and mandrels was that the threaded hole in the mandrel was blind and for manufacturing reasons the thread was kept very short, thus making various lengths necessary to span the range of bone sizes encountered.

The *central bolt* of the TPP exhibited perhaps the most significant modification: the material now used was forged CoCrMo (Protasul-21WF), and the diameter of the shaft was increased from 8 mm to 10 mm. With this material, the risk of fretting and scoring was reduced to a minimum and thus the troublesome chromium plating was abandoned. An increase in shaft diameter called for a corresponding increase in head size, which was now 16 mm (diameter of hemisphere); this in turn called for a larger-sized boss in the *lateral plate*. Apart from this size adjustment, the materials and design of the lateral plate remained unaltered. The hemispherical head of the bolt closely fitted into a bore within the boss of the lateral plate so that, if and when the head lifted off its seat, an axial movement of the bolt of up to 2 mm within the boss was possible while still being radially guided within the bore. As in the prototypes, this was designed to ensure that, even if the bolt became loose through bone remodelling, the TPP would continue to remain constrained within the lateral plate. As previously, a simple locking wire that passed through the bolt head and through slots in the boss of the lateral plate prevented the bolt from turning loose if and when the pre-tension of the bolt dropped off.

In the course of implantation of a total of 64 TPP of this first series (20 in the Orthopaedic University Hospital Balgrist, Zurich, and 44 in the Canton Hospital, Chur), several minor problems were observed. The most annoying step during surgery was probably determining the correct length of central bolt and fitting it. Even though preoperative planning helped to some degree, the final decision could only be made during the operation, and there was often doubt as to whether the bolt had advanced to the end of the blind hole; the bone was therefore not always sufficiently pre-stressed. (A high tightening torque was no guarantee that the thrust plate was being pressed onto the underlying bone).

Another problem which sometimes occurred was due to the rather large-sized boss of the lateral plate, which gave rise to discomfort in patients with little subcutaneous fat; this was especially so if the greater trochanter was so flat that it did not afford much shelter for the lateral plate and bolt head against forces acting on the lateral aspect of the thigh, which tended to irritate the layers of soft tissue in juxtaposition with the plate. Furthermore, a weakness which appeared in five patients in the series was fatigue fracture of the welding joint between the boss and the two straps to which the cortical bone screws were engaged.

Finally, it was generally agreed upon that the circular form of the thrust plate was inappropriate and that it should instead have an oval shape, although no serious problems were observed to have occurred because of this. Only in a few cases with patients of small stature were some transitory complaints noted, especially in the region of the psoas insertion [8]. This modification, together with the introduction of titanium alloy not only for the thrust plate but also for the lateral plate, became the main features of the second series of TPP to be implanted.

Second Series (1988–1991)

As mentioned above, the most significant modifications compared with the first series involved the introduction of titanium alloy for the thrust plate and lateral plate, the two components of the TPP which necessarily were designed to become physically integrated with the living bone. As before, the detailed modifications will be treated taking one component after another, beginning with the thrust plate and ending with the lateral one.

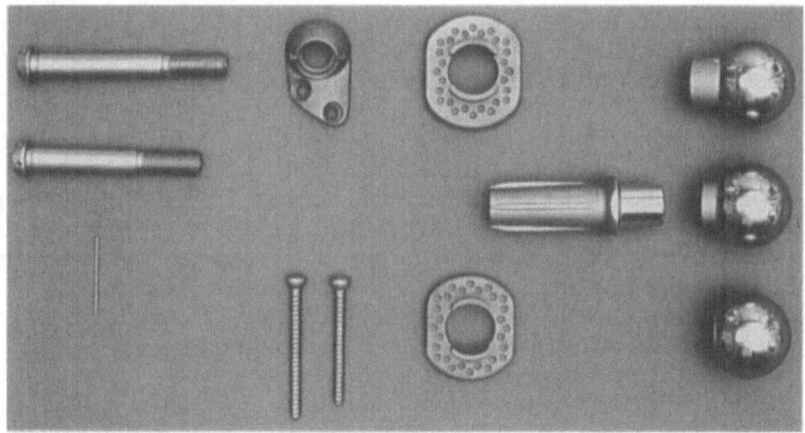

Fig. 9. Components of the thrust plate prosthesis (TPP) of the second series (1988–1991)

Experience and the encouraging results obtained with the first series [8, 9] prompted us to alter the *thrust plate* until it exhibited the form shown in Fig. 9. The plate was no longer circular, but had two segments along its circumference removed so that a roughly oval form resulted. This was closer to the anatomical cross-section of the femoral neck; risk of impingement on the periphery of the acetabular socket in extremes of hip motion could thus be reduced. The surface of the plate that is in contact with the bone was given a similar structure as before, but the peripheral rim which contained the femoral neck was totally eliminated. This led to a greater diameter of the thrust plate of 40 and 44 mm in the two sizes available. The centrally located protrusions, or pedicles, which enter the resected neck were made symmetrical, making it no longer necessary to ensure that the longer protrusion was placed on the side of the calcar. Two grooves and a number of shallow holes in these protrusions afforded additional grip through bone ingrowth; this was particularly necessary at the cranio-lateral aspect of the thrust plate, where, depending on the femoral shaft-neck angle and neck length of the prosthesis, a tendency for the plate to lift off from the bone during gait may be present.

The material chosen was unalloyed titanium. (Four thrust plates of CoCrMo taken from the first series were modified in shape as described above and provided with a plasma-sprayed coating of titanium on the surface in contact with bone. These four were implanted in the Canton's Hospital, Chur in 1985 and 1986). Since the earlier series of TPP showed that on tightening the central bolt the thrust plate often moved slightly relative to the mandrel, adopting a final position that was not exactly normal to the axis of the latter, we decided to retain the spherical shoulder on the mandrel and the corresponding seat in the thrust plate to accommodate for such angular adjustment. Because of this, and in view of the strong tendency for titanium to fret and score under such bearing conditions, it was decided to furnish the thrust plate with a seat insert made of CoCrMo alloy (Protasul-2) that was a shrink fit within the plate.

Extensive tests carried out by the manufacturer and reports in the literature [10] had shown that the combination of CoCr alloys with titanium or titanium alloys is stable and would therefore not give rise to corrosion through galvanic coupling.

The material of the *mandrel* remained cast CoCrMo, but details of the thread for the central bolt were altered. Problems with correct assembly of the central bolt in the first series of TPP strongly advocated the use of a through-hole instead of a blind one. The shaft of the central bolt of 10 mm in diameter continued to be a close fit within the bore of the mandrel, thus making mandrel and bolt one structural unit with virtually no free play between them. As towards the end of the first series, it was considered appropriate to have only one length of mandrel available and to accommodate for various sizes of femora by using a central bolt of appropriate length.

The *central bolt* of the TPP was modified appreciably in this series, not merely with respect to available lengths, but also in connection with the size of head, which had made the boss of the lateral plate unacceptably bulky. The most difficult problem to solve was probably finding a technical solution that offered a small head size with the ability to deviate from the neutral position by about $\pm 15°$ while being constrained radially in a recess (bore) within the boss of the lateral plate together with freedom to move axially lateralwards. A hemispherical head always proved to be too large and therefore could no longer be considered, even though every possible shape of mating boss (which included ones that were partially recessed within the bone) had been taken into consideration. Finally, a practical solution was suggested by M. Imhof of Allo Pro Ltd. in the form of a simple, short, cylindrical head, the head being so short that it could be tilted within the containing bore of the boss by about 10° without jamming. This was by no means an ideal solution, since the slightest deviation of the axis of the bolt from the axis of the bore in the boss causes the head to be tilted against its seat, giving rise to high contact stresses in this area. However, it has always been recognized that the pre-tensioning force of the central bolt is only temporary, lasting for only a few months at the most. This solution was therefore adopted, leaving the material of the central bolt (forged CoCrMo) unaltered. From 1988 to 1991, two lengths of central bolt, 70 and 78 mm, proved to be generally adequate, although a length of 86 mm was also available for special cases.

The *lateral plate* with its boss for accommodating the central bolt was the next item which underwent extensive modification. As it was in intimate contact with cortical bone and was expected to become physically integrated with the underlying cortex, it was agreed that this component should be made of titanium too, as in the case of the thrust plate. To completely eliminate any possibility of strap breakage as encountered in the first series of TPP, we decided to have this made in one piece. Hence the lateral plate now took the form primarily of a boss with a distal plate-like extension that was furnished with two holes for cortical bone screws. The surface of the lateral plate in contact with bone was given a structure similar to that of the thrust plate (several closely set holes of 3 mm in diameter and 0.5 mm in depth); it was also shot-blasted to increase the roughness and thereby further facilitate integration with the underlying bone. To prevent stress shielding of bone, as often encountered under multiple hole plates for osteosynthesis, the distance between the central bolt and the cortical bone screws was kept as short as possible. The bore within the boss that guides the bolt head of 14 mm in diameter was made 4 mm deep so as to permit lateral migration of the bolt head (if this were to occur), while still guiding the bolt radially. It was imperative to allow for this lateral travel in order to guarantee force transmission as envisaged at the proximal end of the femur. The axis of the bore in the boss was at an angle of 115° to the diaphyseal contact surface of the plate; even taking into account the contour of the femur just below the greater trochanter, and in spite of the freedom for angular deviation of the central bolt of about ±10° within the lateral plate, this unfortunately proved to be biased in a varus position. As in the first series of TPP, a simple locking wire was used to prevent rotation of the bolt if it became loose through a drop in pre-tension as a result of bone remodelling.

A total of 102 TPP of this second series were implanted mainly from 1988 onwards, 27 in the Canton's Hospital, Chur, 31 in the Orthopaedic University Hospital Balgrist, Zurich, and 44 in the Clinic for Orthopaedic Surgery, Wattwil. Although implantation was easily accomplished in most cases, some trouble was occasionally experienced with the position taken by the lateral plate on the femur; the plate did not make contact with the bone over any appreciable surface area, the central bolt having already occupied an extreme angular position with respect to the plate so that no further alignment was possible. As pointed out above, this was because of an incorrect angle between bore axis and plate. Because of this, not only did the lateral plate sometimes tend to stand proud of the bone surface at its cranial aspect, but the central bolt became "cocked" in the bore, making tightening difficult, and the problem was accentuated by the scoring that took place under the action of the bolt; this happened when a normal femoral shaft-neck angle of about 130° was maintained, as recommended.

Nevertheless, the early results were even better than those obtained with the first series of TPP, and this finally convinced the manufacturer and supplier to take measures to make this prosthesis available to a wider group of users. In fact, some of the clinical reports presented in this book are a sequel to this effort. Before this had been effected, however, some further modifications to the design had to be carried out in order to correspond to more efficient manufacturing techniques. At the same time, the few problems encountered with the second series were also solved, as reported in detail below.

Third Series (From 1992)

The time had now come not only to reconsider design details in view of more efficient manufacturing techniques, but to also make a final effort to eliminate the few imperfections which were still apparent. Three main modifications were made, one involving the ball head of the prosthesis, another the thrust plate and mandrel and the third the lateral plate of the prosthesis.

From the very start, a ball head with trunnion bearing had been strongly favoured in order to eliminate as far as possible any torque which might occur about the axis of the prosthesis, since this could only be counteracted by the friction between mandrel and thrust plate and by the four shallow ribs on the mandrel that engaged with the surrounding cancellous bone. For strength reasons, the neck diameter of the ball head could not be further reduced, and in order to permit the required range of movement in the hip joint, a head of less than 32 mm in diameter was not possible. By this time, *ball heads* of 28 mm in diameter and corresponding acetabular sockets were being brought on the market, and it was thus considered necessary to take measures to adopt this size of head. We abandoned the 32-mm head of CoCrMo with trunnion bearing for no other reason than this and introduced a 28-mm ceramic head that was attached to the mandrel by a 14-mm *Morse taper*. Since ball heads of ceramic have proved to run very satisfactorily in acetabular sockets of high-density polyethylene (HDPE), we agreed to this change, especially since the 28-mm head was being increasingly demanded. Furthermore, the option of using a 32-mm head was still present, and a 28-mm head of either CoCrMo or ceramic could also be chosen.

The decision to adopt a 14-mm Morse taper on the mandrel for fitting the ball head entailed some alterations to the design of central bolt; there was no longer enough space for the previously employed thread of 10 mm in diameter. Thus we reverted to the 8-mm thread, as used in the prototypes of 1978, but retained the shank or shaft diameter of 10 mm as well as the material of the central bolt (forged CoCrMo) used in the first and second series.

The second major modification involved the *thrust plate* and *mandrel*. To rationalize the manufacturing process, it was requested that thrust plate and mandrel be combined into one component. This was one of the more difficult requests to comply with, since we had on many occasions observed the settling effect of the thrust plate on the resected femoral neck, causing the thrust plate to adopt a final position which was not truly at right angles to the axis of the mandrel. However, since "gap jumping" of bone across gaps of up to 1 mm onto surfaces of bone-inducing materials such as titanium has not only been experienced by us but has also been reported in the literature [11, 12], we rather grudgingly agreed to this modification. Figure 10 shows the thrust plate/mandrel in its present form. Some of the topographical modifications entailed a different profile under the thrust plate and omission of the four shallow ribs, or wings, that ran alongside the mandrel; both were dictated by manufacturing feasibility of the forging die. The thrust plate/mandrel entity, now made of forged TiAlNb alloy, was furnished with a shot-blasted surface to enhance integration with the surrounding bone.

The *central bolt* was basically modified as described above (to adapt to the altered form of mandrel), but its head was also improved by rounding off and polishing the edge of the shoulder that engaged with the seat inside the boss of the lateral plate so as to make tightening of the bolt against its seat easier by preventing scoring of the latter.

Finally, the *lateral plate* itself was corrected so as to more readily achieve the envisaged femoral shaft-neck angle of about 130° by placing the bore in the

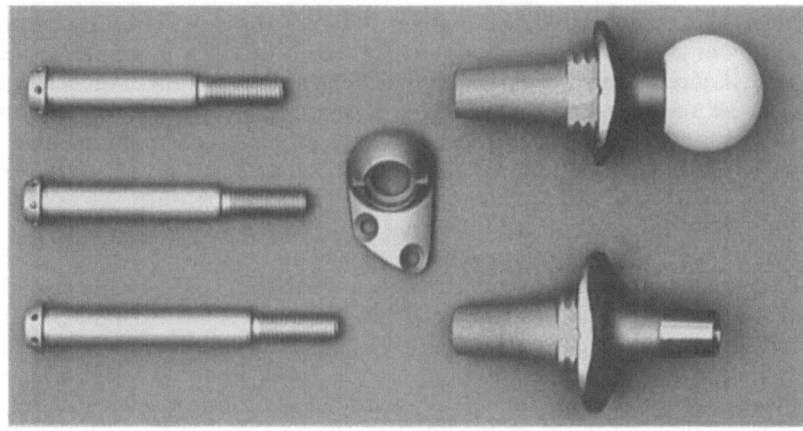

Fig. 10. Components of the thrust plate prosthesis (TPP) of the third series (from 1991 onwards)

boss 5° more in valgus than it had been in the second series of TPP. In addition, to further minimize the tendency for the bolt head to score its seat in the titanium alloy boss on being tightened, the latter has recently (since September 1994) been furnished with an insert made of CoCrMo. A further variation of the lateral plate that has very recently been tested in clinical trials is one made basically of cast CoCrMo but given a plasma-sprayed coating of pure titanium on its underside so as to still ensure bone ongrowth and the desired integration with the underlying bone.

So far, almost 4 years after this third series of TPP was introduced, more than 1500 protheses have been implanted and very satisfactory handling has been reported. The results have continued to remain most encouraging. We have since had the rare opportunity of examining the integration of the titanium thrust plate with the underlying bone on two implants that were removed after some years of service. Although these two cases relate to the second series of TPP, there is no reason why this fortunate finding should not be present in the present series too. More about these two cases is briefly presented below.

Discussion and Conclusions

As described above, the basic concept of the TPP was founded on biomechanical investigations carried out in the 1970s [1, 2], which showed the prime importance of cortical bone in the transmission of mechanical loads. The fact that the cortical bone in the region of the femoral calcar is highly loaded was already shown by Pauwels [13] and has been discussed ever since Wolff's monograph appeared in 1892 [3]. However, we did show that the intramedullarly anchored prosthesis definitely loaded the proximal end of the femur in an unphysiological manner [4], and it was the objective of finding a means of correcting this situation that led to the idea of employing a thrust plate in direct contact with the cortical bone after resection of the femoral neck. It is interesting to note that Philip Wiles [14], who probably developed the world's first total hip prosthesis as early as 1938, also experimented with a design that closely resembles the TPP. This particular design must have been tested in clinical trials in the reported eight cases between the advent of the Judet prosthesis in 1946 and the time of writing in 1957. However, Wiles states that it "was designed to transfer the stress from the cancellous bone of the head of the femur to the dense cortical bone of the shaft", and a radiograph showing this model also indicates that the femoral component of stainless steel was indeed more like a cup that was fitted to the cancellous bone of the head with a straight stem running along the axis of the neck to meet a plate screwed onto the lateral side of the femur. He reported disappointing results, with resorption of bone allowing the stem to slide laterally and project beneath the skin, and therefore abandoned this procedure. If only he had transmitted the hip force directly to the cortical bone!

McKee [15] also experimented in 1950 with a stainless-steel device that had a mandrel running along the neck axis to reach a plate that was attached to the lateral aspect of the femur just below the greater trochanter, but had no plate to transmit the joint force to the resected neck area. In 1957, Picchio [16] used a design resembling that of McKee's but with a collar that was seated on the resected neck. However, the collar showed no design details that would resist the tendency to slip transversally, and the author did not comment on the specific purpose of the collar. In fact, he also showed a prosthesis without a collar. In addition, the cross-sectional drawing of a prosthesis with a collar fitted to the bone shows no differentiation between the cortical and cancellous bone, which possibly indicates that the collar on his prosthesis was not designed to meet the same requirements as the TPP.

The TPP might be characterized by the following properties:

1. The proximal end of the femur continues to be loaded in a physiological manner.
2. By virtue of a pre-stressing arrangement, stability of the prosthesis (immobility with respect to the host bone) is guaranteed immediately after implantation, under normal hip-loading conditions.
3. Due to bone remodelling, pre-stressing of the device against bone gradually drops off in the course of time, but by this time bone ongrowth has advanced to the extent where the thrust plate at one end and the lateral plate at the other have become fully integrated with the living bone.
4. The rigidity of the prosthesis is such that the thrust plate does not tilt away from the underlying bone under the action of hip load.
5. Freedom of the central bolt head to move laterally ensures that the thrust plate always transmits force to the femoral neck. If the bolt head did happen to move, it would continue to be guided by the boss of the lateral plate, thereby preventing the thrust plate from disengaging with the underlying bone by tilting.

6. Since the prosthesis itself lies along just one single axis and has no crank-like offset as in the case of intramedullarly anchored prostheses, it is not subject to any torque.

The above-mentioned properties can of course only be maintained if a few necessary conditions are observed. Firstly, the TPP must be implanted in a correct position, i.e. with a femoral shaft-neck angle of about 130°. A varus position with a femoral shaft-neck angle of less than 120° will probably allow the thrust plate to slowly slip into an increasingly varus position, whereas a valgus position of over 135° will subject the bone to such an unphysiological stress pattern that functional bone adaptation through remodelling will eventually alter the architecture of bone below the thrust plate instead of maintaining it. (Huggler discusses this matter in detail; see Chap. 1, this volume).

Adequate tightening of the central bolt is very important, since only by this means can absolute immobility be obtained. As can readily be appreciated, this is to ensure that no resorption through motion at the bone interface takes place with the formation of soft connective tissue, which would inevitably lead to complete loosening and possibly even to breakage of the implant. The tightening torque is governed by the length of lever arm on the cross-bar of the wrench. No particular torque (Nm) has been specified, since this would encroach on the judgment of the surgeon, who is encouraged to use a high tightening torque according to the given situation. (I am not aware of a single instance in which either the bone was crushed or the bolt thread stripped). In vitro measurements with the 10-mm thread of the first series of TPP showed that the tightening torque is usually about 27 Nm, leading to a pre-compression of the bone of about 8000 N.

The pre-tensioning of the central bolt will gradually diminish. While this is taking place, bone remodelling at the interface is proceeding such that the titanium surface eventually becomes integrated with the underlying bone. This naturally requires bone stock that is capable of undergoing such functional adaptation. As pointed out by Rüther et al. (see Chap. 9, this volume), extensive necrosis of the proximal femur might inhibit such activity in some cases and may thus lead to migration and failure of the implant.

Regarding the stiffness compatibility of the TPP, recent stress analysis computation by the finite element technique has confirmed the basic work done 18 years ago and is presented by Bereiter et al. (see Chap. 3, this volume).

Finally, two rare cases in which the TPP had been removed after an appreciable length of time from patients who had constantly had complaints for unspecific reasons enabled the bone/prosthesis transition to be investigated. Figures 11 and 12 show sections through the specimens (both belonging to the second series of TPP), which were removed 4 and 3.7 years after implantation, respectively. Both clearly indicate the perfect growth of bone onto the titanium surface of the thrust plate without any recognizable soft tissue in between. Also of particular interest are the trajectories of trabeculae that rise to meet the short protrusions of the thrust plate. More about the patient in whom the implant had served for 3.7 years is reported by Schenk et al. (see Chap. 4, this

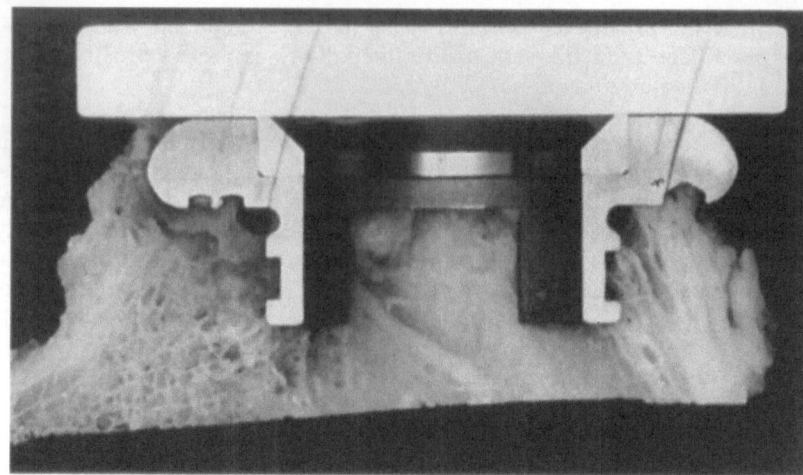

Fig. 11. Male patient born in 1947. Good integration of the titanium thrust plate (second series) with the surrounding bone showing preservation of bone stock in the calcar region after 4 years

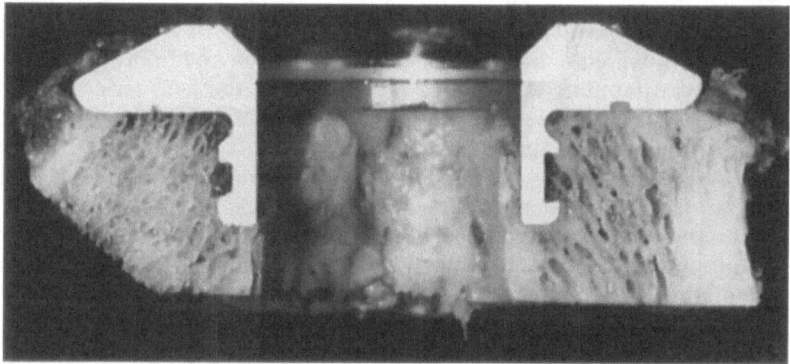

Fig. 12. Patient born in 1939. Excellent integration of the titanium thrust plate (second series) with the surrounding bone showing functional remodelling of the bone, 3 years 8 months after implantation

volume). This, and the encouraging clinical results obtained (reported else-where in this monograph), definitely confirm the sound design and bio-mechanical principles on which this unique hip prosthesis is based.

References

1. Jacob HAC, Huggler AH, Dietschi C, Schreiber A (1976) Mechanical function of sub-chondral bone as experimentally determined on the acetabulum of the human pelvis. J Biomech 9: 625–627

2. Dietschi C (1978) Zur Problematik des künstlichen Hüftgelenkes. Gentner, Stuttgart (Schriftenreihe der MOT, vol 3)
3. Wolff J (1892) Das Gesetz der Transformation der Knochen. Hirschwald, Berlin
4. Jacob HAC, Huggler AH (1980) An Investigation into biomechanical causes of prosthesis stem loosening within the proximal end of the human femur. J Biomech 13: 159–173
5. Weightman B (1976) The stress in total hip prosthesis femoral stems – a comparative experimental study. In: Schaldach M, Höhmann D (eds) Advances in artificial hip and knee joint technology. Springer, Berlin Heidelberg New York, pp 138–147 (Engineering in medicine, vol 2)
6. Semlitsch M (1976) Metallurgical and clinical experience with cast and forged cobalt/chromium base implant metals of compound construction for artificial joint endoprostheses. In: Chapchal G (ed) Reconstruction surgery and traumatology. Karger, Basel, pp 82–101
7. Afifi KF, Jacob HAC (1981) Verschleiss-Messung bei Hüft-Totalendoprothesen mit Polyäthylenpfanne (RCH-1000) und hartverchromtem Protasul-10-Kopf. Z Orthop 119: 157–162
8. Bereiter H, Jacob HAC, Huggler AH (1986) Die klinischen Erfahrungen mit der Druckscheibenprothese. Med Orthop Techn 1: 21–23
9. Schreiber A, Jacob HAC, Suezawa Y, Huggler AH (1983) Erste Ergebnisse mit der sog. Druckscheibenhüfttotalendoprothese (field study). In: Morscher E (ed) Die zementlose Fixation von Hüftendoprothesen. Springer, Berlin Heidelberg New York, pp 134–136
10. Kummer FJ, Rose RM (1983) Corrosion of titanium/cobalt-chromium alloy couples. J Bone Joint Surg 65A: 1125–1126
11. Lintner F, Zweymüller K, Brand G (1987) Histomorphologische Befunde bei zementlos implantierten Titaniumschäften nach mehrjähriger Implantation. In: Refior HJ (ed) Zementfreie Implantation von Hüftgelenksendoprothesen – Standortbestimmung und Tendenzen. Georg Thieme, Stuttgart New York, pp 27–41
12. Schenk RK, Wehrli U (1989) Zur Reaktion des Knochens auf eine zementfreie SL-Femur-Revisionsprothese. Orthopäde 18: 454–462
13. Pauwels F (1965) Gesammelte Abhandlungen zur funktionellen Anatomie des Bewegungsapparates. Springer, Berlin Heidelberg New York
14. Wiles P (1957/58) The surgery of the osteo-arthritic hip. Br J Surg 45: 488–497
15. McKee GK (1967) Developments in total hip replacement. Proc Inst Mech Eng 181: 1966–1967
16. Picchio AA (1960) La ricostruzione dell'articolazione coxo femorale con endoprotesi articolata nella L.C.A. inveterata artrosica bilaterale. Atti del XLV Congresso della Società Italiana di Ortopedia e Traumatologia, Firenze 1960

Finite Element Investigations of the Proximal Femur After Implantation of the Thrust Plate Prosthesis Compared with Findings in a Post-mortem Histological Specimen and in Radiological Follow-Up Examinations

H. Bereiter, M. Bürgi, and R. Schenk

Introduction

Engineered objects can only fulfil their intended function if they exhibit sufficient strength and appropriate deformation and vibration characteristics. This mechanical behaviour is analysed as carefully as possible during the design phase in order to ensure later functional performance. For this, analytical and experimental methods are used.

The value of analytical solutions lies in their transparency, in the possibility to compare alternatives and in the reproducibility of the theoretical model and its assumptions. Analytical models can never exactly replicate real-life conditions. The influence of simplifications and assumptions can, however, be minimized by use of comparative analyses. When doing individual calculations, these influences must be kept as small as possible and quantified by the use of additional experiments.

The idea of dividing up a flat, continuous surface into a number of simply defined elements and obtaining the approximate solution for the whole system from a consolidation of the solutions from the individual elements was first achieved with the force field system and the grid method. The grid method was extended considerably after the introduction of computers, and continua of finite elements became the predominant object of interest. The finite element method has achieved predominance in practice due to its versatility and technical transparency, offering the following possibilities:

- Complicated geometry, loading patterns, associated factors and clamping conditions present no particular problems in the development of models and in numerical processing.
- Material properties such as modulus of elasticity or changes to it as a result of loading can be assigned to each element as needed.
- The properties at the connection between individual elements can be defined as desired [11].

The finite element (FE) method was introduced into biomechanics in the 1970s [9]. It dealt in particular with the deformation behaviour of bone with and without an endoprosthesis. Knowledge gained from similar work considerably influenced the further development of implants [5, 10].

A hip-joint prosthesis changes the loading on the bone considerably. The most common prosthesis models are now stem prostheses with intramedullary fixation. The thrust plate prosthesis (TPP) differs fundamentally from these in that it attempts to transfer the forces resulting from the joint via a thrust plate directly onto the femoral neck. The objective is to take full account of the morphological bone structure. Thus it is attempted to obtain bone loading in the proximal femoral area which is as close to the physiological condition as possible [3].

In hip-joint endoprosthetics, the clinical results alone are only of limited value because they usually only appear much later than the radiologically determined changes in the bone. Precise radiological follow-up analyses are generally able to detect a loosening problem or a prospective implant failure much earlier. Even better evidence is provided by histological investigations on cadaveric specimens, which permit quantitative and qualitative judgements to be made concerning the reaction of the bone to the implant and vice versa [2, 8].

Based on the finite element method, this chapter examines the changes in bone loading and the resulting deformation behaviour following implantation of a TPP and compares these with the results to date from radiological follow-up examinations and with a histological specimen.

Materials and Methods

The loading of the healthy implant-free bone during the one-legged stance in walking, taking into account investigations by Pauwels, served as the basis for further calculations on bone with an implant.

This loading condition was also the basis for the investigation of the TPP without bolt pre-stressing, which might be assumed to follow bone remodelling.

Material Properties, Geometry of the Femur and Loading

The material properties of cortical and cancellous bone were taken from a review of the literature [1, 4, 6]. The cortical bone was defined as transverse isotropic material. The cancellous bone was divided into several areas with different orthotropic material properties. For the calculations for the femur with an implant, an approximation was used with a mean modulus of elasticity of the cancellous bone remaining after resection, because the greatest differences in the moduli lie in the resected parts.

The inner and outer surfaces of the femoral cortical bone were in the form of boundary curves which were developed from computer tomographic sections of a cadaveric femur.

The previously noted loading model according to Pauwels was defined as follows for the loading case: a resulting tensile load of 1300 N on the trochanter major in the frontal plane, inclined 25° medially; a compressive load of 1750 N on the ball head, applied at 20° in the lateral and 5° in the dorsal direction.

Proximal End of the Femur Without Implant

In order to be able to compare the calculations for various implants, calculations were carried out for healthy bone without an implant. The femoral model comprises 3700 nodes and about 3200 volume elements. In order to avoid excessive distortion of elements, the trochanter minor could not be modelled to its full height. The cortical bone is extremely thin in the area of the trochanter major and the caput femoris and has little influence on the bone load-carrying behaviour. Moreover, the zones that were important for our investigation do not lie in these areas. The model that was used therefore ignores this thin cortical layer.

Proximal End of the Femur with the Thrust Plate Prosthesis

The models consist of approximately 7000 nodes and 5500 volume elements. In the remodelled condition, it is assumed that there is solid mechanical fixation in the region of the pedicles. In the case of the thrust plate, the contact zone is simulated using compression elements, because in tension, ongrowth cannot be simply assumed (Fig. 1).

Histological Autopsy Specimen

A proximal section of a femur with a thrust plate still in place was retrieved during autopsy from an 87-year-old woman; the TPP had been in situ for 8 years and had not given rise to any clinical problems. The patient weighed 55 kg and had normal mobility until the time of death.

The specimen removed post-mortem had indicated adequate bone remodelling conditions radiologically. Radiographs of the contralateral hip that had been furnished with a conventional cemented prosthesis 4 months after the TPP had been implanted indicated bone resorption processes in the area of the medial cortical bone of the femoral neck (Fig. 2).

Following appropriate preparation, the specimen with the thrust plate was sawn in various planes so that a histological investigation in the important loading areas was possible. Bone staining was done using toluidine. With this stain, older bone appears blue, while new, young bone appears dark violet (Fig. 3).

Radiography

The radiological follow-up examinations were performed using standard techniques. Additional anteroposterior (AP) shots were taken with 20° inward rotation in order to have the bone contact surface of the thrust plate parallel to the axis of radiography. A correct AP picture of the proximal femur was thus possible, avoiding misinterpretation otherwise due to the antetorsion of the femoral neck.

Fig. 1. Finite element (FE) model with
an implanted thrust plate prosthesis
(TPP)

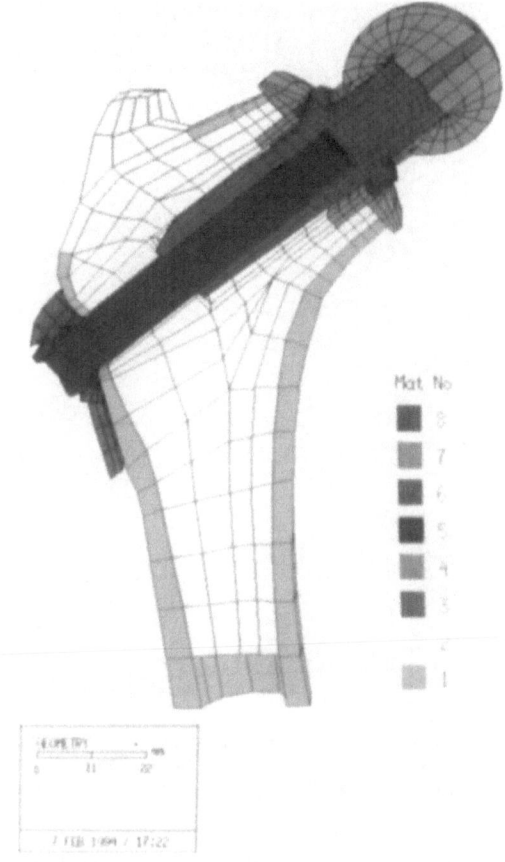

Results

Finite Element Calculations

The calculations using the finite element method showed that the deformation of the proximal femur under load occurs continuously from proximal to distal.

In the AP projection, the femur is deformed in the medial direction. Where a conventional cemented stem prosthesis is implanted, the model shows a stiffening of the proximal femur, and the main deformation takes place distal to the stem. With the TPP, however, the deformation behaviour under load is practically identical to the normal femur (Fig. 4).

With a stem prosthesis, the von Mises stresses occurring in the loaded cortical bone show a clear reduction in the area of the proximal femur. With the TPP, however, the stress pattern is practically the same as with a normal femur under load (Fig. 5).

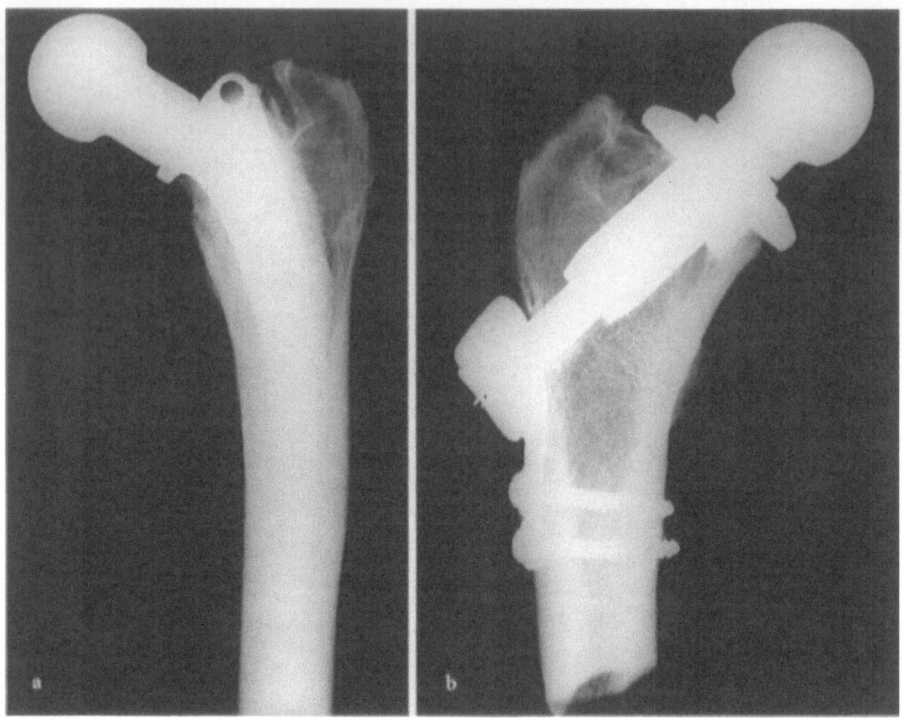

Fig. 2a,b. Radiographs of post-mortem explants. **a** Conventional cemented prosthesis. Resorption of the medial cortical bone of the femoral neck. **b** Thrust plate prosthesis (TPP) with normal radiological conditions and retention of cortical bone in the femoral neck

Only in the cancellous bone of the caudal femoral neck, at the level of the so-called pedicles, are higher stresses than in the normal femur observed (Fig. 6).

Histology

The complete histological view in section 1 shows that the cortical bone of the medial femoral neck is strong and formed normally. There is no osseous contact on the cranial side of the thrust plate. In contrast, there is direct osseous contact on the caudal side. The area of the so-called pedicles, in particular, exhibits direct ongrowth of bone. Fresh bone is also detectable, giving wide support to the chromium-cobalt thrust plate. The bone loss directly medial under the thrust plate is caused by destructive polyethylene granuloma. The lateral plate and the associated screws are stable and have firm mechanical fixation in the bone (Fig. 7).

In sections 2 and 3, ventral and dorsal to the medial frontal plane of the femoral neck, the bone under the thrust plate shows large areas of growth onto the metal. The visible gaps are artefacts from the histological preparation.

Fig. 3. Section planes 1–3 of the histological investigations of the femoral neck

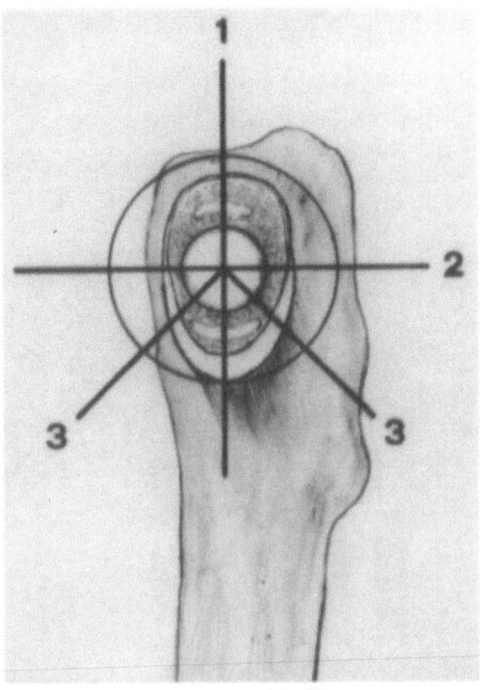

Here, the bone exhibits a peduncular support reaction and consists mainly of cortical components. The trabeculae leading away underneath exhibit an ordered structure which appears to be remodelled according to the applied load (Fig. 8).

Radiology

The radiological follow-up examinations of patients without problems 12, 10 and 2 years after implantation show good retention of the femoral neck cortical bone. Indications of atrophy or unfavourable bone restructuring are not visible. Under the thrust plate, adaptive remodelling is found in the femoral neck cortical bone and at the level of the pedicles in the form of bone density increase and oriented new trabecular structures with a corresponding supportive reaction (Fig. 9).

The results of the analyses clearly show that the deformation behaviour and stress distribution in the proximal end of the femur following implantation of a TPP is scarcely different from that in the normal physiological state. The histological investigations confirm the direct ongrowth onto the thrust plate, with osseous structures adapted to the loading pattern. Radiologically, the cortical bone of the medial femoral neck retains its function. Additionally, the follow-up examinations indicate an increase in osseous structures underneath the thrust plate and a little distal from it, at the level of the so-called pedicles.

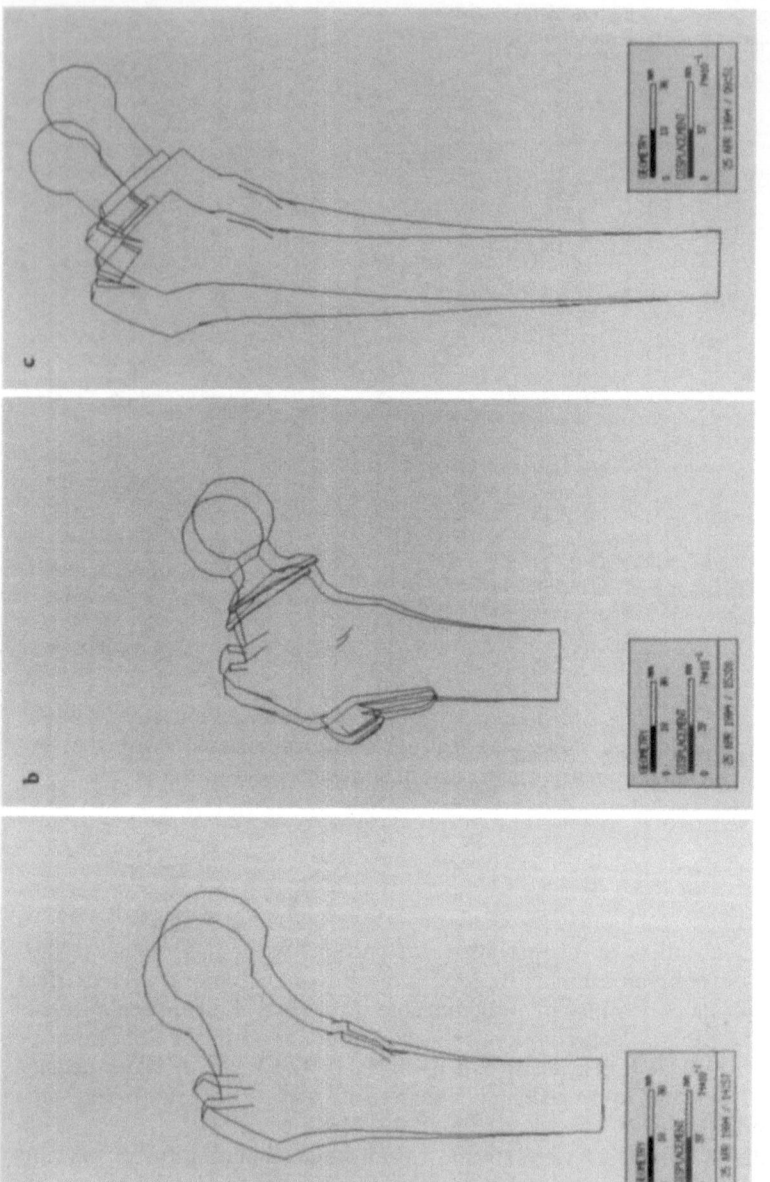

Fig. 4. a Deformation behaviour of the normal femur. **b** Deformation behaviour of the femur with an implanted thrust plate prosthesis (TPP). **c** Deformation behaviour of the femur with a conventional cemented prosthesis. The calculated deformations show that there is great similarity between a normal femur and a femur implanted with a TPP. However, a conventional cemented stem prosthesis stiffens the proximal end of the femur, and deformation occurs mainly in the distal area in the region of the diaphysis

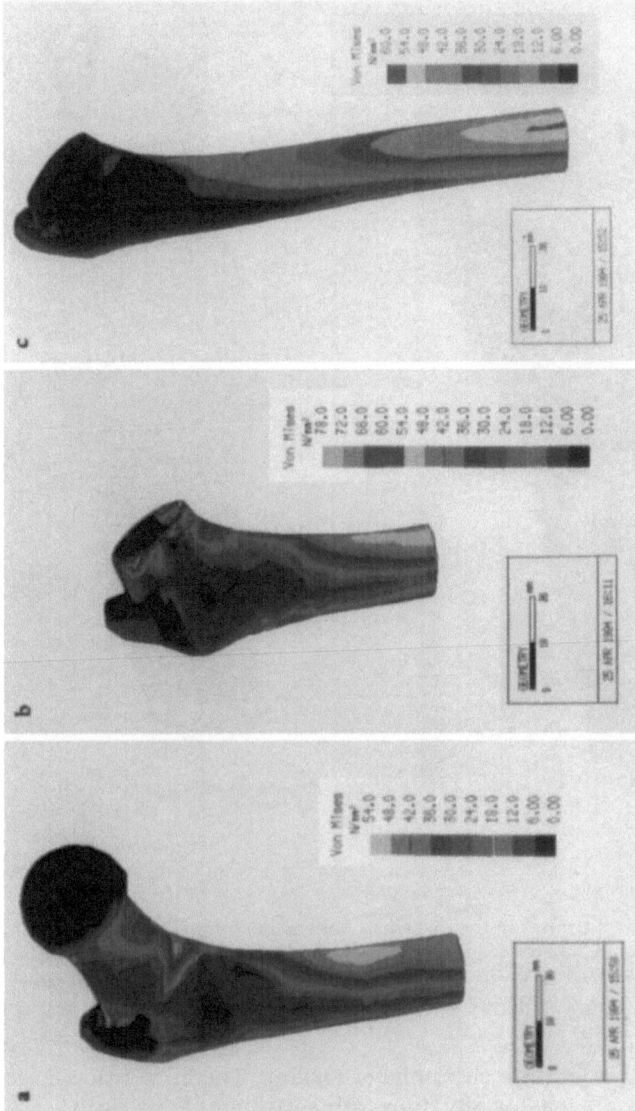

Fig. 5. a Von Mises stresses in the proximal cortical bone of a normal femur. **b** Von Mises stresses in the cortical bone with an implanted thrust plate prosthesis (TPP). **c** Von Mises stresses in the cortical bone with an implanted cemented stem prosthesis. The von Mises stresses in the proximal femur under normal conditions are very similar to those with the implanted TPP. With a conventional cemented stem prosthesis, there is significant stress relief of the proximal femur, especially in the medial region of the femoral neck

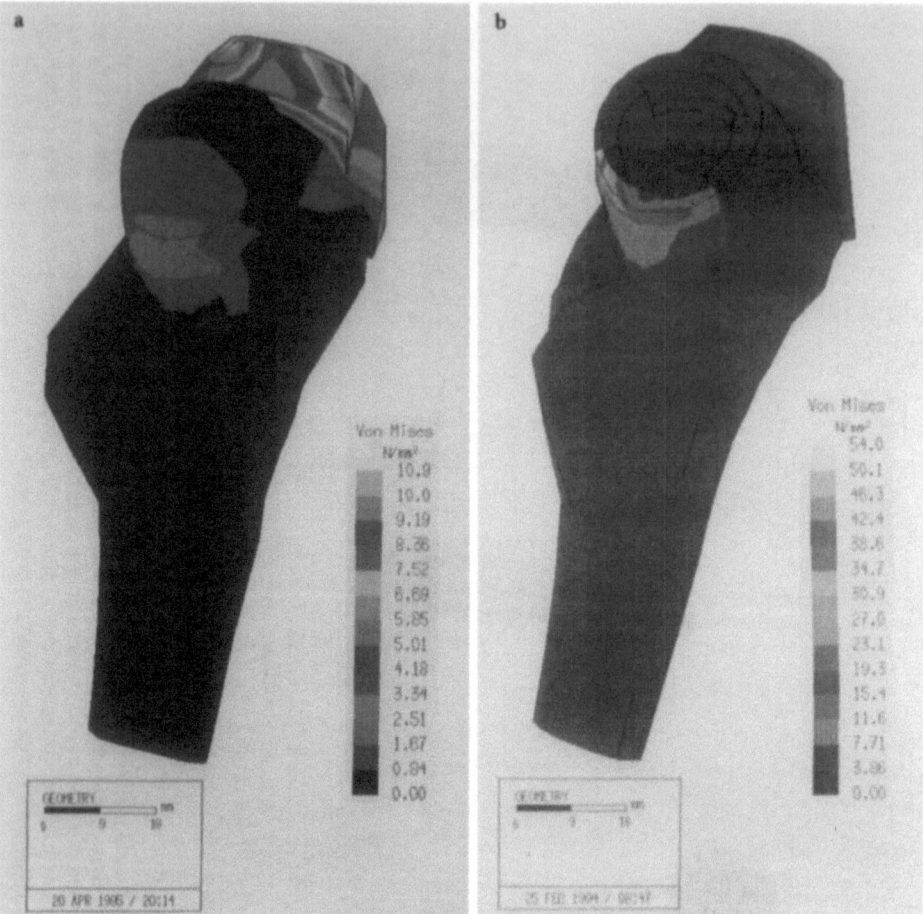

Fig. 6. a Von Mises stresses in the cancellous bone of the normal femoral neck (caput femoris resected). **b** Von Mises stresses in the cancellous bone with an implanted thrust plate prosthesis (TPP). The loading of the cancellous bone directly caudal beneath the disk and at the level of the pedicles is increased compared with the normal condition

Analyses of this location show higher loading. The bone reacts in this region adequately to the loading situation with corresponding growth.

Discussion

The basic concept involved in the TPP as a hip-joint implant is the transfer of the forces from the joint directly onto the medial cortical bone of the femoral neck. An attempt is thus made to closely correspond to anatomical and morphological factors. The TPP is therefore an implant with extramedullary fixation and direct load transfer onto the femoral neck. As a result, all the

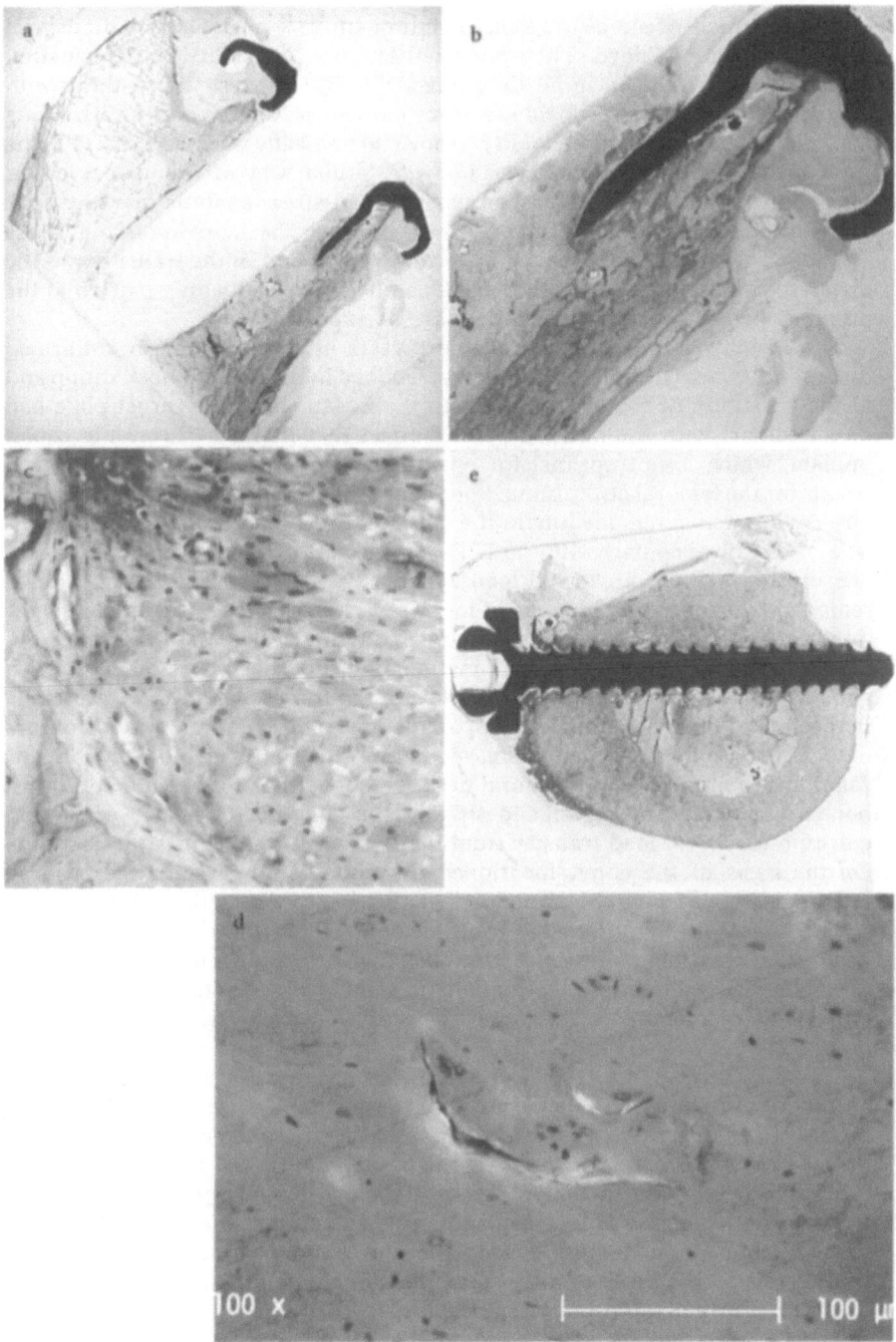

Fig. 7. a Complete view of section 1. The quality of the medial cortical bone of the femoral neck has been retained. Proximal to this region there is no contact with the thrust plate. **b,c** Bone loss due to polyethylene granuloma. **d** Polyethylene particles in the region shown in b in polarized light. **e** Integration of the lateral plate screws

problems which occur as a result of intramedullary metaphysial–diaphysial load transfer are avoided. These include basic non-physiological deformation and stress pattern for the bone. Compared with the TPP, a stem prosthesis with intramedullary fixation probably requires more bone remodelling effort. Using the finite element method, it could be shown analytically that, with the TPP, the proximal end of the femur behaves in a very similar way to the normal femur. This confirms the results of earlier experimental stress analysis investigations as reported by Jacob (see Chap 2, this volume). The corresponding stress distribution in the femoral neck, in the metaphysis and in the transition to the diaphysis are maintained. With the TPP, a physiological loading pattern at the proximal end of the femur may therefore be expected.

The histological specimen available 8 years after implantation confirmed these conditions. The bone structure was retained in the femoral neck stump and in the transition of the femoral neck to the metaphysis. The thrust plate had direct contact with the bone, despite the fact that it was a chromium-cobalt implant, which is not optimal for osseointegration. Similar to the analytical results for the femoral neck stump, bone adaptation and new bone growth can be observed as active remodelling in the areas of direct load transfer. The peduncular direct bone contact with the TPP and the underlying trabecular structures are adapted to the transferred loads. Increased bone growth and favourable remodelling is observed in areas of increased stresses. Optimum osseointegration of the implant with remodelled bone structure is therefore exhibited.

The radiological follow-up examinations indicate that where the TPP has a good fit, additional bone apposition beneath the thrust plate occurs, especially in the area of the medial pedicle. Apparently a greater compressive load occurs here. Calculations show that increased compressive stresses do occur in this cancellous bone area of the femoral neck. The bone thus reacts with additional bone apposition in this region and supports the TPP. The trabecular orientation corresponds to the load transfer from the implant to the femoral neck stump. On the basis of the above-mentioned osseointegration, we may also speak radiologically of favourable functional adaptation to the loading situation.

The histologically observable zones of bone resorption directly medial beneath the thrust plate are caused by polyethylene wear granuloma. However, 8 years after implantation, the granuloma activity is restricted to a very small area in the medial area of the femoral neck, while corrective bone activity is observable at the same time.

Since 1992, the Ti-6Al-7Nb forged alloy Protasul-100 has been used with a 12/14 taper spigot in the TPP design, thus permitting the use of the Metasul all-metal articulation, which reduces the risk of particle-induced granuloma.

In summary, it can be stated that the basic concept and functioning of the TPP have been confirmed not only analytically, but also histologically and radiologically. The physiological loading pattern and the osseous structures are retained. Bone remodelling is adequate and is adapted to the loads being transferred. In the areas of direct load transfer at the implant–bone interface, direct bone contact and bone remodelling adapted to the stresses can be observed [2, 7, 8, 10]. The same conditions are present in the area of increased stress in the cancellous bone of the femoral neck, where the formation of new

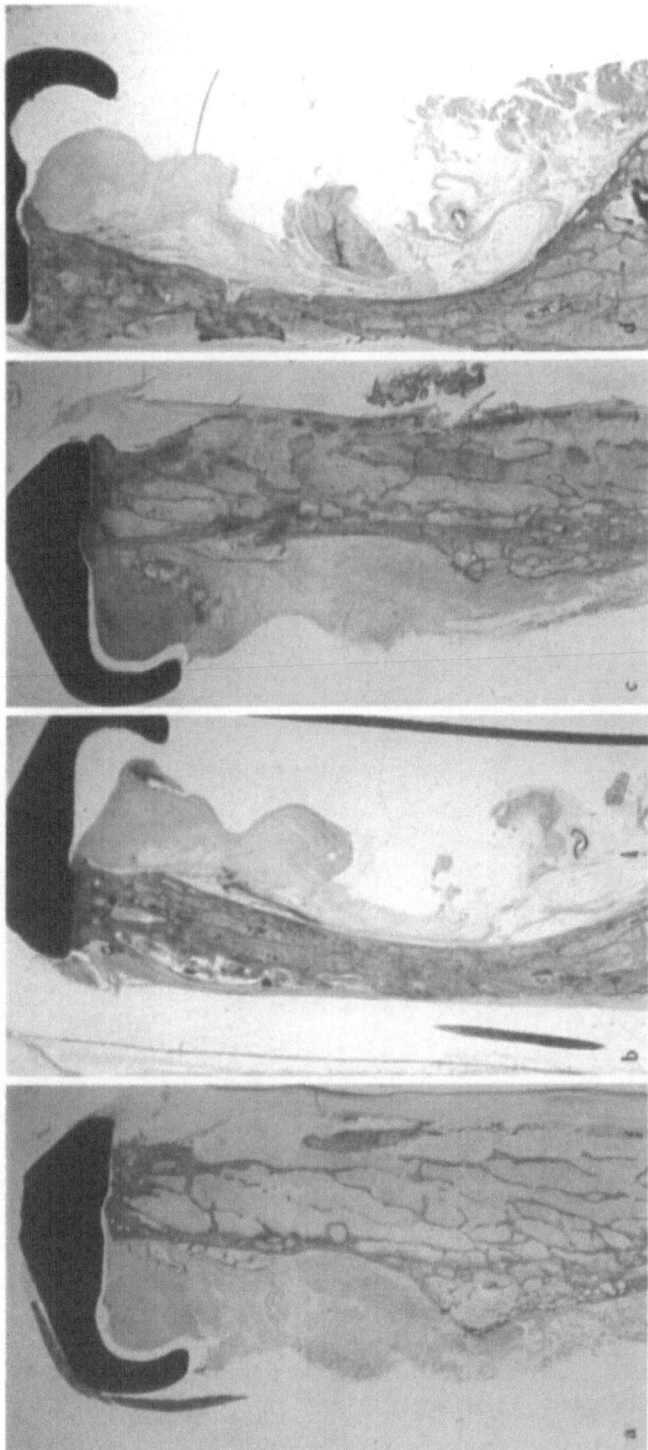

Fig. 8a,b. Section 2 through the femoral neck ventral and dorsal. **c,d** Section 3 through the femoral neck ventral and dorsal. Noteworthy is the good bone support directly beneath the thrust plate in the form of strong peduncular cortical support with direct apposition on the thrust plate. The underlying osseous trabeculae have adapted to the load. **e–h** Enlargement of the area directly under the thrust plate prosthesis in sections 2 and 3. The gap is an artefact caused by the machining process during the histological preparation. Direct bone contact with peduncular support reaction and load-oriented trabecular structures can thus be confirmed

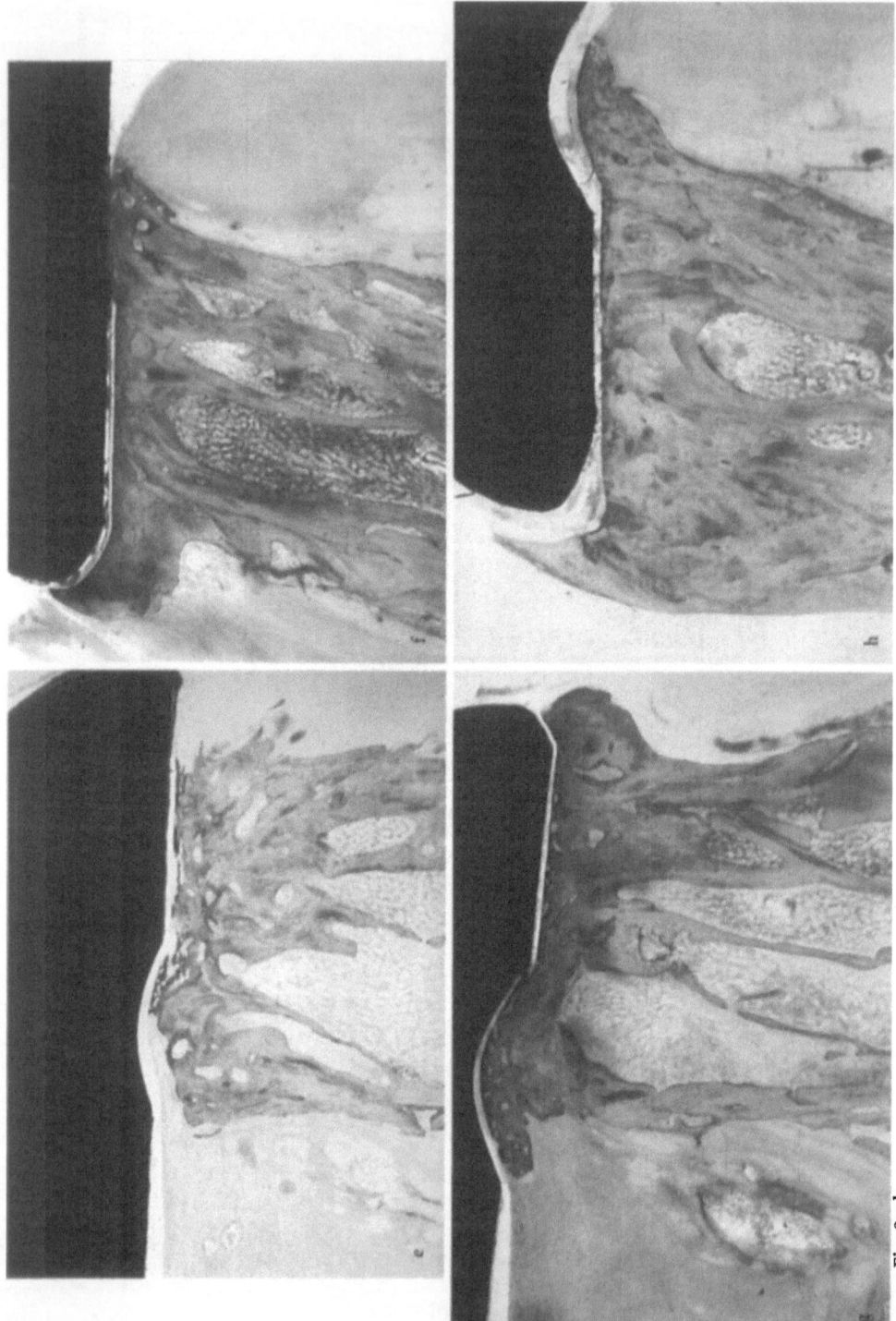

Fig. 8e–h

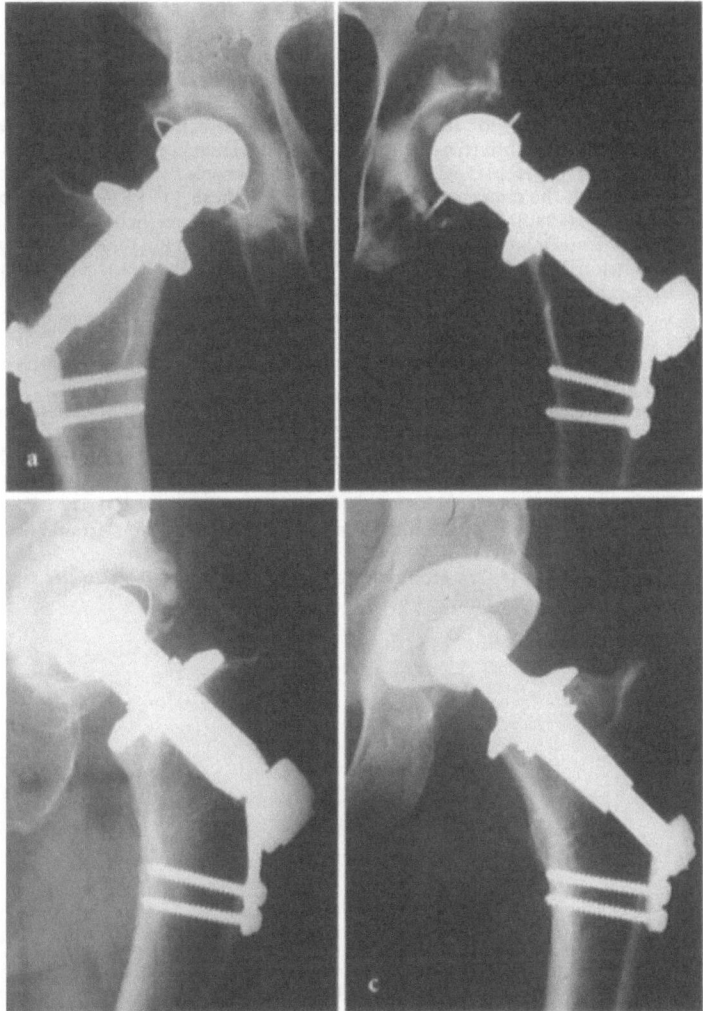

Fig. 9. a Result after 12 years with a thrust plate prosthesis (TPP); female patient operated on both hips within 3 months. The patient is subjectively pain-free and completely mobile. Very good bone structure is visible in the area of the medial cortical bone of the femoral neck, without any bone resorption. **b** Results after 10 years; very well retained medial cortical bone of the femoral neck is visible. Especially visible in this female patient is the additional reactive bone growth directly under the TPP, directed towards the so-called pedicles of the disk. **c** Result after 2 years of the definitive design using titanium alloy. Here, too, the increase of structured bone under the thrust plate at the level of the pedicles can be observed

trabeculae adapts to the loading, and increased bone density is observed. The concept of the TPP represents an interesting alternative to previous hip implants with intramedullary fixation.

References

1. Asman RB, Cowin SC (1984) A continous wave technique for the measurement of the elastic properties of cortical bone. J Biomech 17 (6): 349–361
2. Bereiter H, Bürgi M, Rahn BH (1992) Das zeitliche Verhalten der Verankerung einer zementfrei implantierten Hüftpfanne im Tierversuch. Orthopade 21: 63–70
3. Huggler AH, Jacob HAC, Bereiter H, Haferkorn M, Ryf C, Schenk R (1993) Long-term results with the uncemented Thrust Plate Prosthesis (TPP). Acta Orthop Belg 59 [Suppl 1]
4. Knauss P (1980) Materialkennwerte und Festigkeitsverhalten des spongiösen und kompakten Knochengewebes am koxalen human-Femur. PhD thesis, University of Stuttgart
5. Middleton J, Nade GN, Williams KR (1992) Recent advances in computer methods in biomechanics and biomedical engineering. Walters, Swansea
6. Reilly DT, Burstein AH (1975) The elastic and ultimate properties of compact bone tissue. J Biomech 8: 3393
7. Schenk RK (1991) Reaktion des Knochens auf Implantate. In: Stuhler T (ed) Hüftkopfnekrose. Springer, Berlin Heidelberg New York, pp 533–558
8. Schenk RK, Wehrli U (1989) Zur Reaktion des Knochens auf eine zementfreie SL-Femur-Revisionsprothese. Orthopadie 18: 454–462
9. Scholten R (1975) Über die Berechnung der mechanischen Beanspruchung in Knochenstrukturen mittels für den Flugzeugbau entwickelte Rechenverfahren. Med Orthop Tech 6: 130–137
10. Weinans HH (1991) Mechanically induced bone adaptations around orthopaedic implants. Haveka, Ablasserdam
11. Zienkiewicz OC (1977) Methode der finiten Elemente, 3rd edn. Hanser, Munich

CHAPTER 4

Histology of the Thrust Plate–Bone Interface

R.K. Schenk, R. Hauser, A.H. Huggler, and H.A.C. Jacob

Introduction

A thrust plate prosthesis (TPP) implant of the second generation was removed after 3 years and 8 months due to pain and functional impairment of unknown origin. The thrust plate was made of titanium with a rough, shot-blasted surface (see Chap. 2). The thrust plate–bone interface was subjected to a histological examination as follows.

Case Report

A male patient, born in 1939, suffered from slowly increasing pain and functional impairment of his right hip over a period of 7 years. In 1984 X-rays revealed an osteoarthritis due to an epiphysiolysis of the femoral head. The disabling condition and severe pain remained unresponsive to repeated conservative treatment performed until 1991. An advanced secondary osteoarthritis grade III was diagnosed at the Orthopaedic University Clinic in Zurich, where the decision for a hip replacement in the form of a TPP was made and carried out in April 1991. Peri- and postoperative measures included prophylactic medication with Mandokef (cephamandole). The intervention as well as the postoperative rehabilitation were uneventful. Three months after the operation, the patient complained again of pain at the site of the scar, on weight-bearing. Sitting or walking were also painful, while pain during night rest depended on the positioning of the right leg. Poor gait and hip function due to this pain in the hip as well as in the right ankle, where a post-traumatic arthritis was diagnosed, led to the patient being unable to work (taxi driver).

At the follow-up examination in 1994, the patient showed a slight tenderness at the medial aspect of the scar, a Duchenne limp and painful rotational movements of the right hip. The patient was again hospitalized. Blood chemistry and X-rays showed no signs of infection.

In December 1994, the patient underwent hip revision under peri- and postoperative Mandokef medication. The operation revealed a local bursitis at the site of the lateral plate. The thrust plate was firmly seated on the femoral neck. The acetabular socket was stable. Four bacteriological samples (socket, femoral neck, lateral plate) were removed for investigation. The examination showed staphylococcus coagulase negative in the region of the lateral plate (bursitis) whereas the femoral neck area appeared inconspicuous.

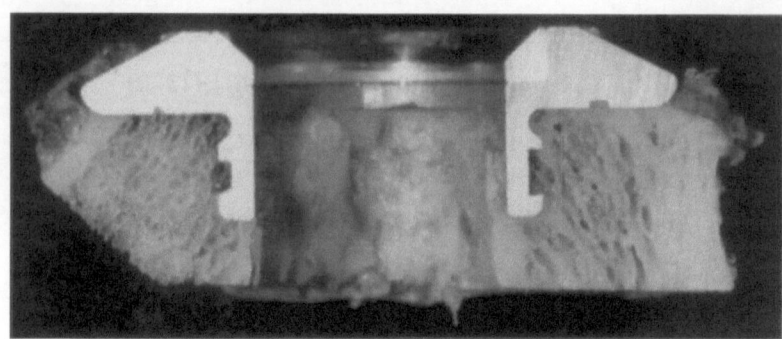

Fig. 1. The dorsal half of the thrust plate–bone specimen after division in the frontal plane

The polyethylene inlay of the Balgrist metal-backed socket was replaced and a cementless intramedullarly anchored Zweymüller prosthesis with a 28 mm head implanted. Under postoperative long-term antibiotics (Augmentin, amoxicillin) the patient recovered without functional disability and with no pain.

Material and Methods

On revision, the femoral neck was osteotomized at a distance of about 12 mm in a plane parallel to the bearing surface of the thrust plate. The interface between the plate and its bony support thereby remained intact, and the bone around the pedicles (see Chap. 2) was therefore fully preserved. A closer inspection of the specimen revealed an excellent coverage of plate and supporting bone in the superior, anterior and inferior segments, whereas the posterior margin of the plate extended beyond the periosteal surface of the femoral neck. After fixation in neutral, buffered formalin, the specimen was split in the frontal plane with a thin carborundum abrasive disc, and photographs of the cut surfaces were taken (Fig. 1). Inspection with a stereo microscope indicated extensive and intimate bone-implant contact that could be successfully preserved during the following steps of dehydration, infiltration, and final embedding in methyl methacrylate.

Fig. 2a–c. Frontal section of the superior part of the middle portion of the thrust plate. Ground section, surface staining with toluidin blue and basic fuchsin. a Two compact bony struts converge towards the superior margin of the plate and the distal rim of the pedicle. The remaining surface of the implant is supported by cancellous bone. Bone is also deposited in the space between the pedicle and the mandrel (arrow). b The superior strut consists of regular cortical bone and still undergoes intensive remodelling. Pre-existing bone appears lighter (arrow). c Newly formed compact bone embodies the bulgy distal rim of the pedicle. Perfect contact and continuing remodelling along the bone-implant interface

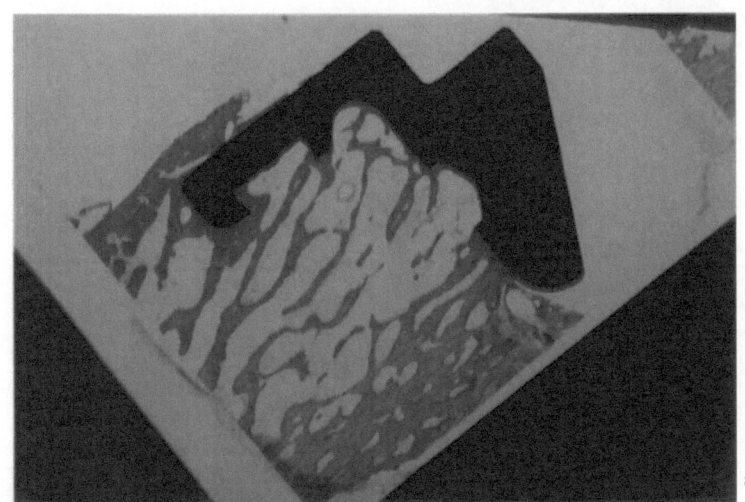

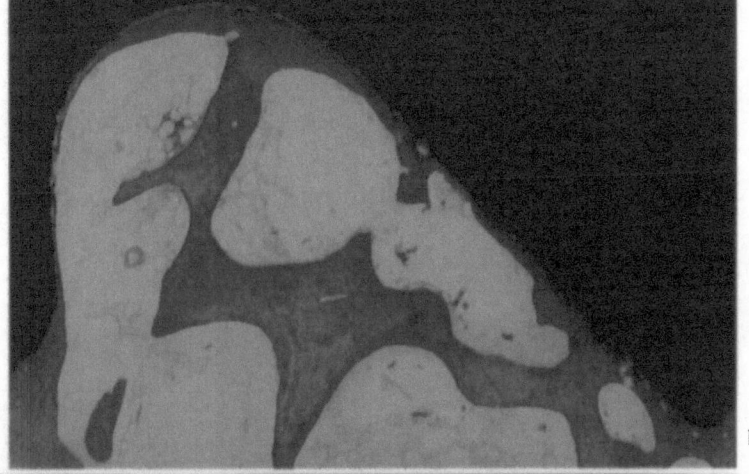

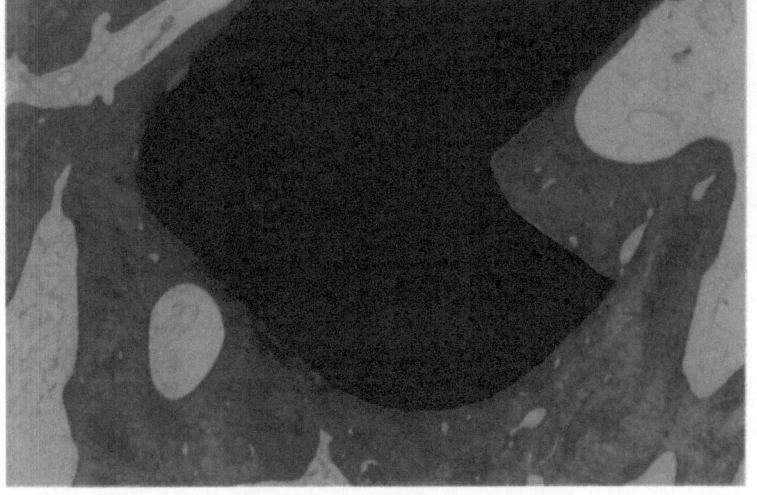

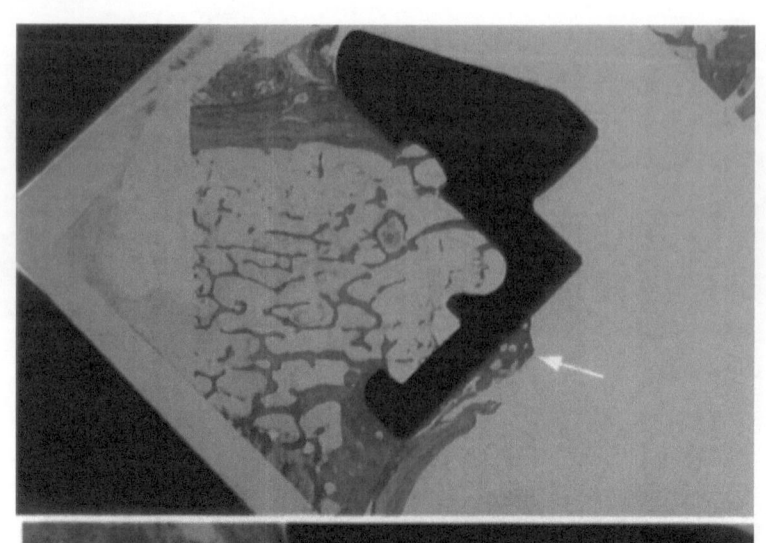

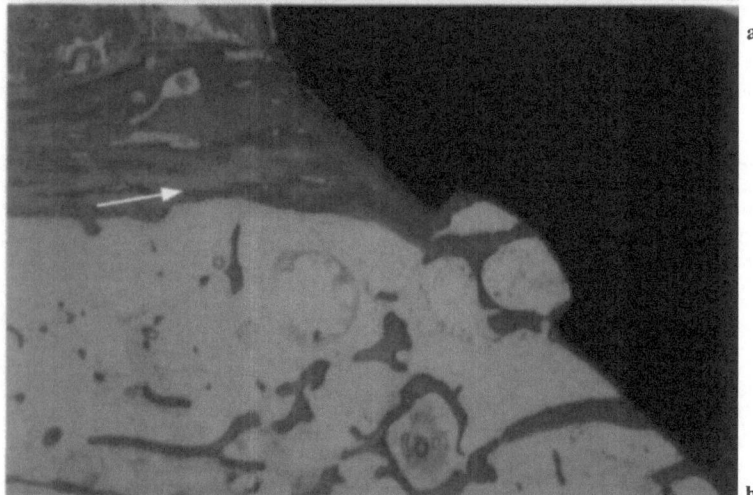

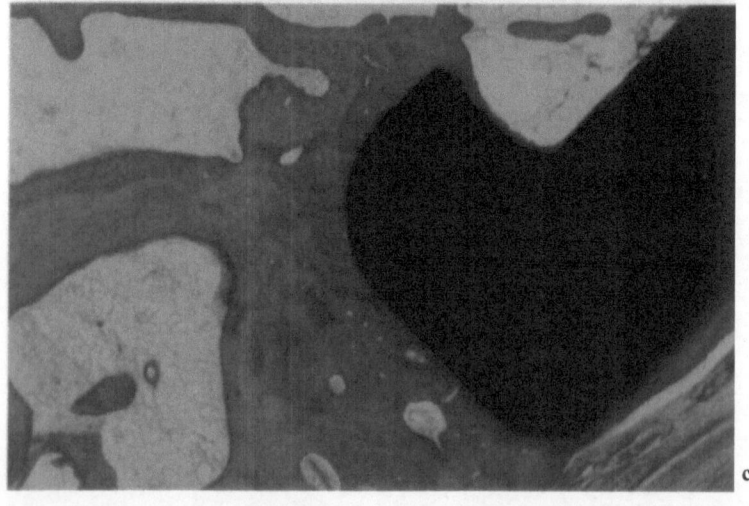

From both blocks, 0.5–0.7 mm thick sections were cut with a diamond wafering blade, starting from the frontal surfaces exposed during the preparation. The sections were glued to opaque plexiglass plates of common slide format (5×5 cm), ground and polished to a final thickness of 80–100 μm, and surface stained with toluidin blue, or toluidin blue and basic fuchsin [1]. The posterior block was cut all the way through in the frontal plane (Figs. 5, 6), whereas, after taking frontal sections (Figs. 2, 3), the anterior block was finally cut perpendicular to this plane for better visualization of the anterior support (Fig. 4).

Microscopic Observations

Frontal Sections of the Middle Portion

The microphotographs of these specimens are all oriented in a position that shows the thrust plate at an inclination of 45° to the sagittal plane. This corresponds to the common orientation of the femur in routine anterior–posterior radiographs. All frontal sections comprise both the superior and the inferior segments of the thrust plate together with the respective pedicles (see Chap. 2), separated by the space originally occupied by the mandrel. The surfaces in direct contact with the implant surface facing the bone and bone marrow of the femoral stump are preserved (Figs. 2a, 3a). Vigorous bony struts rise up to meet the margins of the plate as well as the distal bulge of the pedicles.

In the superior portion (Fig. 2a) a cortical plate supports the margin and extends in a horizontal position towards the trochanter area. Microscopically, this strut includes remnants of the original cortical layer, reinforced and partially substituted by new osteons (Fig. 2b). The remodelling activity in this area is remarkably high. The bone near the interface is thoroughly viable, and consists mainly of primary and secondary osteons. Another compact strut supports the distal rim of the superior pedicle and runs almost parallel to the axis of the femoral neck. It encompasses the distal rim of the pedicle with a thick layer of newly formed bone (Fig. 2c) which contains few remnants of preexisting, and now devitalized trabeculae. The superior portion of the area in between the bony anchors contains cancellous bone of relative low density. The trabeculae are preferably oriented in a horizontal direction and make localized contact with the titanium surface (Fig. 2a,b).

◄───

Fig. 3a–c. Frontal section of the inferior part of middle portion of the thrust plate. Ground section, surface staining with toluidin blue and basic fuchsin. **a** Structural organization analogous to Fig. 2, but different orientation of the trabeculae in the cancellous compartment which closely resembles the **physiological architecture of the calcar area**. **b** The angle between plate and pedicle is supported by the thickened end of trabeculae which fuse with the continuous bony coating along the rough titanium surface. **c** The bony incorporation of the pedicle rim is symmetrical to the superior counterpart (Fig. 2c)

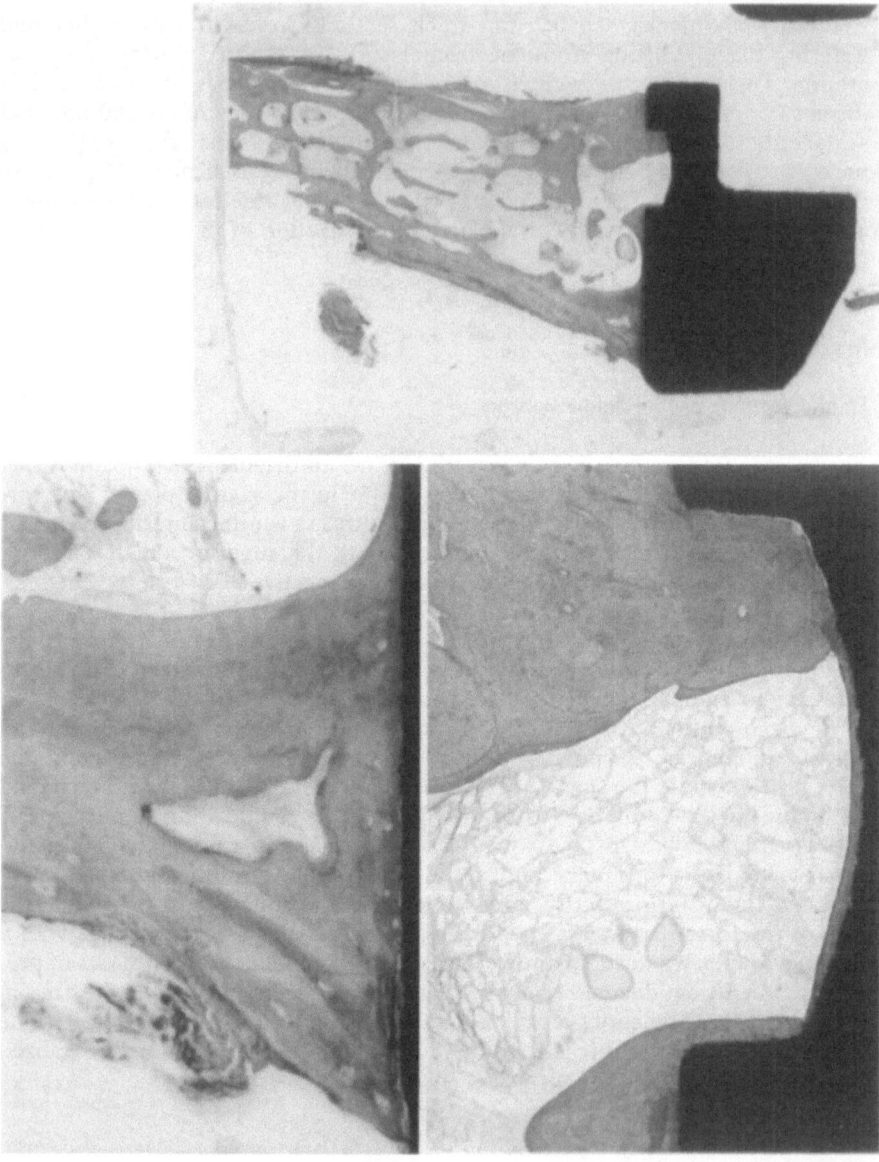

Fig. 4a-c. Transverse section of the anterior portion of the thrust plate. Ground section, surface staining with toluidin blue and basic fuchsin. **a** The anterior and posterior portions are not furnished with pedicles. The bony support concentrates again upon the periosteal and newly formed inner cortical layer, suplemented by some trabeculae in the interzone. **b** The subperiosteal cortical layer contacts the implant surface through a compact, fully regenerated layer. Nonviable remnants of preexisting osteons again appear lighter than the surrounding regenerated bone. **c** Higher magnification of a pit, showing a 50 μm thick bony coating of the tough titanium surface. The margins of the pit are supported by vigorus lamellar bone struts

The inferior portion presents a similar structural organization (Fig. 3a). The cancellous portion exhibits a higher overall density. This spongiosa consists of plates, partially bifurcating or interconnected by transverse septa. The trabeculae converge towards the protruding elements of the implant surface, where they are firmly anchored. In between the terminations of the trabecular struts, a continuous, thin layer of lamellar bone covers most of the titanium surface (Fig. 3b). Again, the bulgy rim of the pedicle is surrounded by a deposit of viable compact bone (Fig. 3c). Bone was also deposited within the slot between the pedicle and the mandrel, both in the superior and inferior sectional planes (Figs. 2a, 3a).

Sections Through the Anterior Portion

After cutting the frontal sections, the anterior block was reoriented and transverse sections of the anterior portion were made (Fig. 4). This part of the thrust plate is not furnished with pedicles, but exhibits on its flat inner surface circular pits measuring 2–3 mm in diameter. Again, the bony support bears mainly upon the margins of the plate. The subperiosteal support consists of cortical bone. Some of the preexisting cortex is preserved, but has undergone extensive remodelling and reinforcement by apposition of lamellar bone (Fig. 4b). The cancellous bone facing the mandrel is also transformed into a cortical layer which bears the inner margin of the plate. The space in between these cortical layers is occupied by cancellous bone. Some trabeculae contact the inner aspect of the implant, mainly the edges and protruding elements. In addition, the flat parts, as well as the walls of the pits are almost completely lined by a sheet of lamellar bone, measuring about 50 μm in thickness (Fig. 4c). As in the frontal sections, the titanium surfaces are in contact with regenerated, viable bone. Areas of primary contact between metal and preexisting devascularized bone are extremely rare.

Sections Through the Posterior Part

The whole posterior block was sectioned in the frontal plane. Macroscopic inspection already revealed that the bone support of the posterior margin of the plate was incomplete and overhung the posterior periosteal envelope of the femoral neck. A slightly oblique transitional section (Fig. 5a) still includes the inferior pedicle, which is encompassed by solid compact bone (Fig. 5c). Most of this area, however, rests upon dense connective tissue, representing the periosteum and remnants of the original joint capsule and ligaments. The superior portion is supported by cortical and cancellous bone beyond its full extent (Fig. 5b). The pits have been filled with bone, and the cortical areas exhibit a remarkably high remodelling activity.

In one of the last sections of this frontal series (Fig. 6a), the bony support is restricted to the superior area of the posterior margin of the plate. The bone-implant interface is still intact, and bone has invaded the pits (Fig. 6b). The

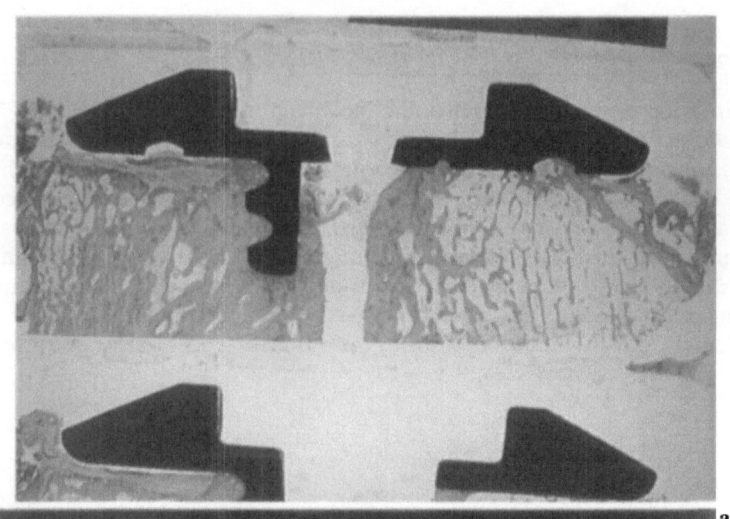

a

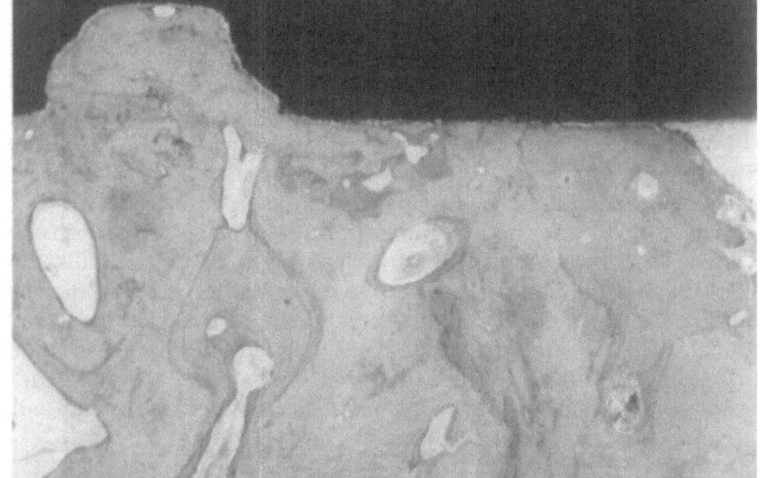

b

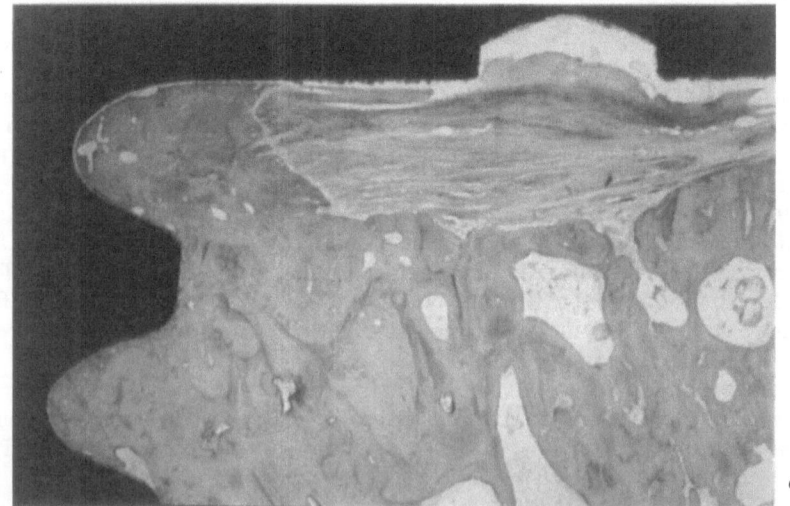

c

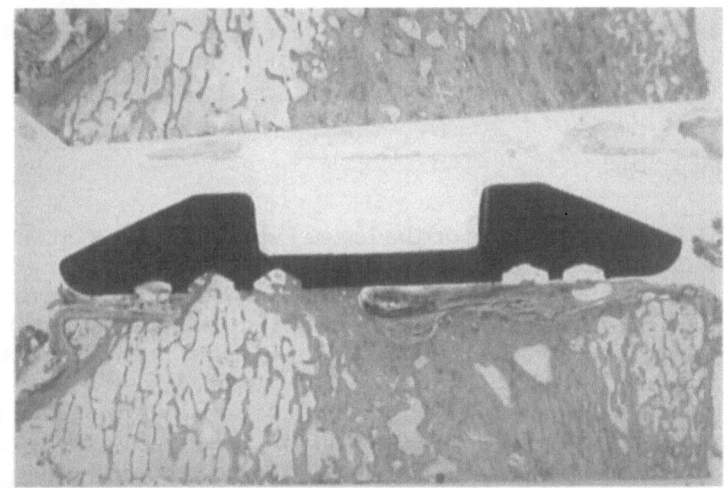

a

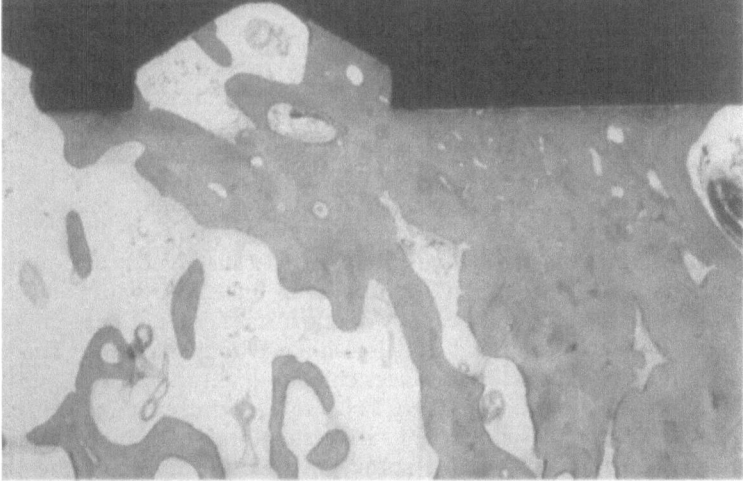

b

Fig. 6a,b. Frontal section through the posterior portion of the thrust plate. Same orientation as Fig. 5. Surface staining with toluidin blue and basic fuchsin. a Bony support is restricted to the superior part, whereas the inferior part (*to the right*) is lined by connective tissue. b Towards the center, compact bone still supports the implant. The excellent bone quality and the perfectly intact bone-implant interface proves stability and osseointegration

◀

Fig. 5a–c. Frontal, slightly oblique section of the transitional zone between the middle and posterior portion of the thrust plate. a The inferior part (*to the right*) still carries the marginal portion of the pedicle. It is only partially supported by bone. The superior part (without pedicle) is again supported by cortical bone which concentrates upon its margins. Surface staining with toluidin blue. b Bone-implant interface of the inner pillar. Toluidin blue clearly stained the cement lines which illustrate the ongoing and past remodelling activities. c The pedicle is completely encompassed by lamellar bone. The remaining inner aspect of the plate is lined by dense connective tissue, stemming from the original periosteum and joint capsule

inferior part is separated from the bone by the interposition of dense fibrous tissue which again represents the periosteum and remnants of the former capsule.

Discussion

Osseointegration in its original sense means bony incorporation of cementless implants, achieved by direct bone deposition upon the implant surface [2]. This first step is followed by functional adaptation of the surrounding bone to the local loading conditions by changes in bone mass and structure. The histological mechanism of osseointegration shares many characteristics with direct or primary fracture healing, and accordingly can be subdivided into three overlapping stages [3]: (1) initial stabilization by woven bone formation, (2) adaptation of the bone mass to load by reinforcement with lamellar bone, and (3) adaptation of the bone structure to load by cortical and trabecular remodelling. The first stage dominates within the first 4–6 weeks, the second stage begins at 1–2 months, and remodelling becomes effective after 3–5 months. The adaptational processes continue over years, or even lifelong. The first and second stage of osseointegration are decisive for the incorporation of the implant in its bony surroundings.

Besides the need for precise fitting and primary stability to be achieved at implantation, bony incorporation depends mainly on material properties. Commercially obtainable pure titanium and titanium alloys are now widely accepted as materials with excellent tissue compatibility. Bony ongrowth, which can be taken as a measure of the so-called osteophilic properties, is not only favoured by the material properties, but also by the fine structure of the implant surface. In this respect, rough surfaces do not only improve adhesion of the bone to the surface, but also enhance bony ongrowth. The superiority of titanium plasma sprayed surfaces compared to machined or polished titanium was already described in 1976 [4]. More recently, animal experiments have shown that rough, sandblasted surfaces might even be more attractive for bone deposition than the plasma spray [5], besides improving the shear strength between implants and bone [6]. In histological studies of femoral stems retrieved at autopsy, the excellent osteophilic properties of rough blasted titanium surfaces could also be demonstrated [7, 8]. In this study it could be shown that bone ongrowth is not limited to those areas where forces are transmitted (bony anchors), but extends even upon surface areas which are apparently not exposed to mechanical load. This "bony coating" with less than 50 μm thick lamellar bone suggest that rough titanium surfaces might directly stimulate osteogenesis by undifferentiated bone marrow stroma cells.

With an implantation period of 3 years and 8 months, this specimen clearly falls into the third stage of osseointegration. Successful osseointegration is proven by the perfect contact along the bone–implant interface. There are no interpositions of connective tissue nor fibrocartilage which would indicate a localized microinstability, nor any deformations of the bone matrix structure that could result from local overload. Moreover, the bone adjacent to the contact areas is viable, and inclusions of dead fragments along this borderline are extremely rare. This is the result of direct lamellar bone apposition (during stage 2) and/or remodelling (stage 3) that has accomplished substitution of avascular areas produced at surgery. Localized reinforcements of the more compact bony anchors, as well as the architecture of the trabecular framework in the cancellous parts also suggest that functional adaptation, commonly explained by Wolff's law, is almost completed. These histological observations, therefore, confirm the mechanical concepts that have lead to the design of the thrust plate in its current form.

Summary

A thrust plate made of titanium was retrieved at revision after 3 years and 8 months and was thoroughly examined in undecalcified histological sections. The findings confirm perfect osseointegration. Direct contact with viable bone was found along all the implant surfaces facing the bone and bone marrow, and subsequent modelling and remodelling activity has selectively reinforced and structurally adapted the load bearing cortical and trabecular compartments.

References

1. Schenk RK, Olah AJ, Herrmann W (1984) Preparation of calcified tissues for light microscopy. In: Dickson GR (ed) Methods of calcified tissue preparation. Elsevier, Amsterdam, pp 1–56
2. Brånemark P-I, Hansson BO, Adell R, Breine U, Lindström J, Hallen O, Oemann A (1977) Osseo-integrated implants in the treatment of the edentulous jaw. Experience from a 10-year period. Scand J Plast Reconstr Surg [Suppl] 11
3. Schenk R (1995) Osseointegration of Sulmesh Coatings. In: Morscher EW (ed) Endoprosthetics. Springer, Berlin Heidelberg New York, pp 60–71
4. Schroeder A, Pohler O, Sutter F (1976) Gewebsreaktion auf ein Titan-Hohlzylinderimplantat mit Titan-Spritzschichtoberfläche. Schweiz Monatsschr Zahnheilkd 86: 713
5. Buser D, Schenk RK, Steinemann S, Fiorellini JP, Fox CH, Stich H (1991) Influence of surface characteristics on bone integration of titanium implants. A histomorphometric study in miniature pigs. J Biomed Mater Res 25: 889–902
6. Wilke HJ, Claes L, Steinemann S (1990) The influence of various titanium surfaces on the interface shear strength between implants and bone. In: Heimke G, Soltész U, Lee AJC (eds) Clinical implant materials. Elsevier, Amsterdam, pp 309–314 (Advances in biomaterials, vol 9)
7. Schenk RK, Wehrli U (1989) Zur Reaktion des Knochens auf eine zementfreie SL-Femur-Revisions-Prothese. Orthopäde 16: 454–462
8. Spotorno L, Schenk RK, Dietschi C, Romagnoli S, Mumenthaler A (1987) Unsere Erfahrungen mit nicht-zementierten Prothesen. Orthopäde 16: 225–238

The First-Generation Thrust Plate Prosthesis: Long-Term Results of a Clinical Pilot Study of 20 Cases

R. HAUSER and T. KUHN

Introduction

At the end of the 1970s Huggler and Jacob developed a hip endoprosthesis with a new concept for femoral fixation, aiming at a physiological transfer of load from the femoral component to the proximal femur [2]. The first generation of this thrust plate prosthesis (TPP) was implanted in the Canton Hospital, Chur, Switzerland, from 1978, and in the Balgrist Orthopaedic University Clinic, Zurich, Switzerland, from 1980 onwards.

The long-term results of the TPPs implanted in Chur have already been published [1]. The objective of this chapter is to present the results of the TPPs implanted in Zurich in 1980 and 1981. The ethics committee of the hospital permitted an initial implantation of a series of only 20 TPPs and required that the decision as to whether this prosthesis concept could be considered for further implantations be made on the basis of long-term clinical results. This cautious evaluation of a new prosthesis design was the object of this clinical pilot study, which is recommendable for every new development, but is scarcely ever carried out.

Material and Method

In the period from 1 October 1980 until 3 April 1981, 20 TPPs were implanted in 19 patients in the Balgrist Orthopaedic University Clinic in Zurich. In one patient both hips were operated on. Of the 19 patients 15 were men and 4 women. The average age at operation was 54.9 years (range 77–35). The etiology of the 20 treated hip disorders was as follows: 11 cases of idiopathic coxarthrosis and 9 cases of femoral head necrosis (5 idiopathic, 2 posttraumatic, 2 as a result of metabolic disturbances). In 8 hips there had been a previous surgical intervention: 7 cases of intertrochanteric osteotomy and 1 case of osteosynthesis following femoral neck fracture.

The first-generation TPP was manufactured completely from a cobalt-chromium alloys (Fig. 1). A 32-mm diameter modular rotational head was used throughout. The acetabular component was a cemented polyethylene socket in all cases. The operations were carried out by two surgeons, with 18 TTPs implanted by the more senior one. The average duration of the operation was 91 min (65–200 min).

Fig. 1. The first-generation TPP in cobalt-chromium alloy and with a 32-mm rotational head

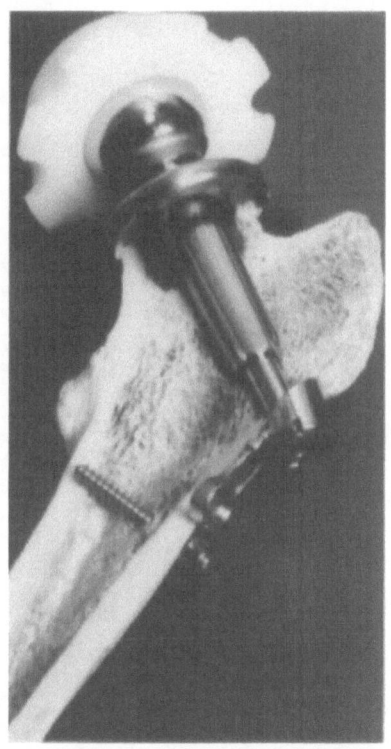

Routine follow-up examinations of all patients were carried out annually. Figure 2 shows the follow-up periods for all 20 cases. Due to reintervention the revised TPPs obviously have limited follow-up. In the 15 TPPs in which no revision operation is known, six have a follow-up period of less than 10 years. Three of these six patients have died, and the other three were lost to follow-up as the patients are foreigners who returned to their native country.

The results are presented in the form of a survival analysis. The radiological findings and the clinical results are also presented.

Results

No intraoperative complications occurred during implantation of the 20 endoprostheses. In the early postoperative period in one case a pulmonary embolism was suspected.

In the following period 5 of the 20 prostheses had to be revised due to loosening. Acetabular and femoral components were revised in all cases. The two earliest revision operations, after 7 and 10 months respectively, were due to septic loosening. The three other revision operations, after 24, 113, and 131 months, respectively, were due to aseptic loosening. The survival curves (Ka-

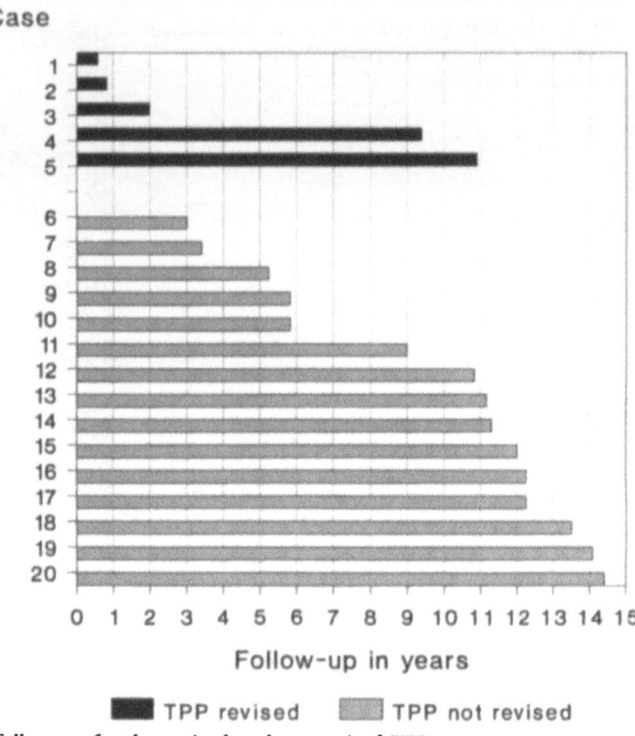

Fig. 2. Description of the follow-up for the revised and nonrevised TPPs

plan-Meier) are shown for the two different failure criteria. Figure 3 shows the survival curve based on failure of all five revision operations (septic and aseptic loosenings). Figure 4 shows the survival curve based only on the criterion of aseptic loosening.

Table 1 gives the values of the survival time analysis (life table method) of the survival curve as shown in Fig. 3, which considers all 5 revised prostheses. The 10-year survival rate, including the revision operations for septic and aseptic loosening, is 77.6%. When the criteria failure include only the revision operations due to aseptic loosening, 10-year survival is 86.2% (Table 2).

The following four parameters were investigated in the radiological analysis and measured in millimetres (Fig. 5): Osteolysis line proximal (a) and distal (b) to the mandrel of the TPP; the caudolateral shift of the central bolt out of the lateral plate (z), and the thickness of the medial cortical bone (d) halfway between the seated thrust plate and the beginning of the trochanter minor. The correlation between the clinical condition and these radiological findings indicated that a caudolateral shift of the central bolt out of the lateral plate (z) of up to 4 mm over the course of 10 years is not necessarily associated with discomfort or with other radiological signs of loosening (Fig. 6). It was also established that a thin radiological osteolysis line of up to 4 mm in the upper area of the mandrel (a) does not necessarily cause pain or other detrimental

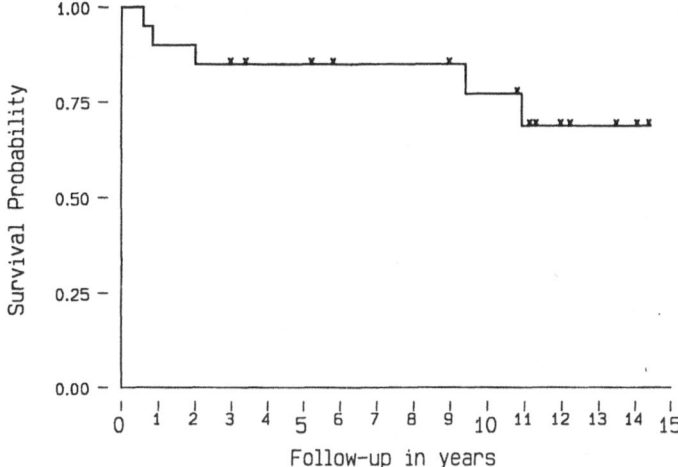

Fig. 3. Survival curve (Kaplan-Meier) of 20 TPPs. The failure criterion is the revision operation ($n=5$) due to septic ($n=2$) and aseptic ($n=3$) loosening

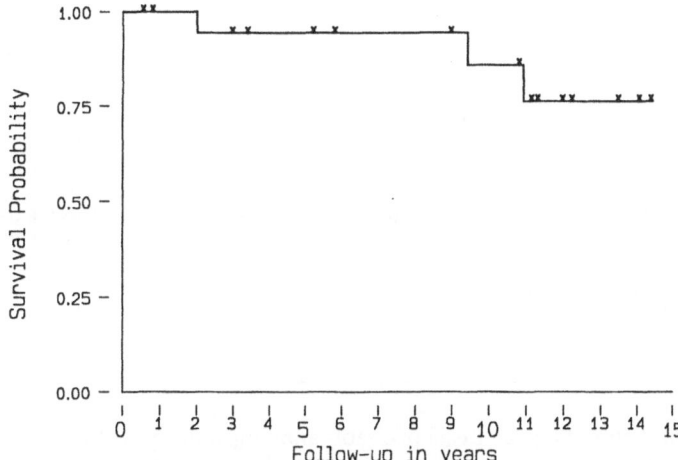

Fig. 4. Survival curve (Kaplan-Meier) of 20 TPPs. The failure criterion is the revision operation ($n=3$) due to aseptic loosening ($n=3$)

conditions in the long term. Based on these observations, the following radiological criteria for prosthesis loosening were established: Radiologically, a TPP may be considered as being loose when the sum of caudolateral shift of the central bolt (z) plus the osteolysis line in the proximal area of the mandrel (a) is greater than 8 mm. Using this criterion, 3 of the 15 TPPs that were not revised must be considered radiologically to have been loose. In these cases there was also slight osteolysis in the distal area of the mandrel (b), an in-

Table 1. Survival time analysis [life table method; failure criterion: revision operation ($n=5$) due to septic ($n=2$) and aseptic ($n=3$) loosening]

Interval since operation (years)	Number of prostheses followed at start of interval	Failed (revised prostheses)	Withdrawn	Estimated rate not to fail (survival probability)	95% CI	
0–1	20	2	0	0.900 ± 0.067	0.656	0.974
2–3	18	1	0	0.850 ± 0.079	0.603	0.949
3–4	17	0	2	0.850 ± 0.079	0.603	0.949
5–6	15	0	3	0.850 ± 0.079	0.603	0.949
9–10	12	1	1	0.776 ± 0.101	0.498	0.911
10–11	10	1	1	0.694 ± 0.119	0.399	0.865
11–12	8	0	2	0.694 ± 0.119	0.399	0.865
12–13	6	0	3	0.694 ± 0.119	0.399	0.865
13–14	3	0	1	–	–	–
14–15	2	0	2	–	–	–

Table 2. Survival time analysis [life table method; failure criterion: revision operation ($n=3$) due to aseptic loosening ($n=3$)]

Interval since operation (years)	Number of prostheses followed at start of interval	Failed (revised prostheses)	Withdrawn	Estimated rate not to fail (survival probability)	95% CI	
0–1	20	0	2	1.000 ± 0.000		
2–3	18	1	0	0.944 ± 0.054	0.666	0.992
3–4	17	0	2	0.944 ± 0.054	0.666	0.992
5–6	15	0	3	0.944 ± 0.054	0.666	0.992
9–10	12	1	1	0.862 ± 0.092	0.541	0.964
10–11	10	1	1	0.771 ± 0.119	0.433	0.922
11–12	8	0	2	0.771 ± 0.119	0.433	0.922
12–13	6	0	3	0.771 ± 0.119	0.433	0.922
13–14	3	0	1	–	–	–
14–15	2	0	2	–	–	–

dication of a prosthesis probably moving slightly within the femoral neck. Four of the 12 TPPs classified as absolutely radiologically stable show none of the above radiological changes (a, z).

In none of the cases did the thickness of the medial cortical bone (d) decrease. There was an increase of more than 2 mm in the thickness of this medial cortical bone in more than half of the nonrevised TPPs. Significant osteolysis or defects of the proximal femur at the level of the TPP were not observed. Based on a qualitative estimate, a slight, scarcely noticeable eccentric wear of the polyethylene socket was observed in all cases. In none of the 15 nonrevised cases was there an indication that the polyethylene socket had loosened.

A clinical rating was carried out using the Harris hip score (Fig. 7). This is shown separately for the two groups – radiologically loose and radiologically

Fig. 5. Scheme of the four radiologically analyzed parameters

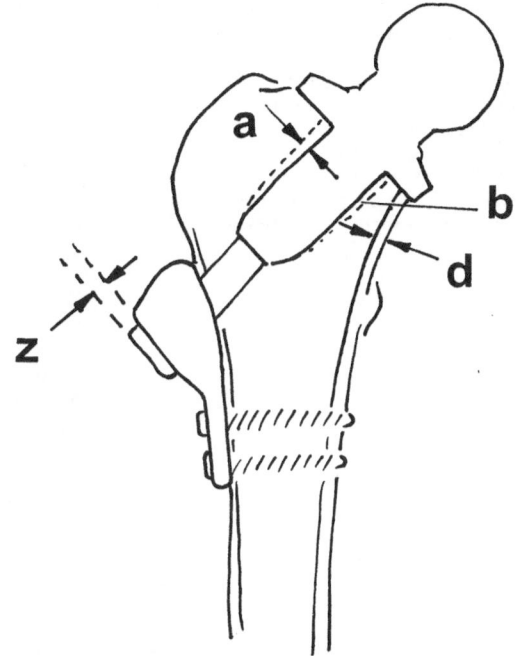

stable. A TPP classified as radiologically loose with a hip score of 85 can be categorized clinically as good, and a radiologically nonloosened TPP with a score of 42.5 can be categorized as very poor. In this latter case the significant pain was due to severe periarticular ossification.

The patients themselves assessed their condition with the artificial joint as follows: In the group of 12 TPPs classified as stable, 8 patients were "very satisfied," two were "for the most part satisfied," one was "partly satisfied," and one was "unsatisfied." In the group of three prostheses classified as loosened, one patient each was "very satisfied," "partly satisfied," and "unsatisfied."

A total of five complications of mechanical nature were recorded. In three cases the lateral plate fractured, in one case associated with an aseptic loosening of the femoral component. In the other two cases the fracture of the lateral plate had no negative effects, and the prosthesis was classified as radiologically stable in the long-term. In two cases the central bolt was changed after 4 years and freshly tightened. In one case the progression of radiological loosening could not be halted. In the other the TPP was stabilized by tightening the bolt, and the Harris hip score at the last follow-up examination was 83 points.

Discussion

Defining a revision operation as a failure criterion due to septic or aseptic loosening, 10-year survival with the TPP was 77.6%. Considering only the cases

Fig. 6a–c. Radiological follow-up of a TPP. **a** Initial finding with severe coxarthrosis and a slightly dysplastic acetabulum. **b** Radiograph immediately following the implantation of a cemented polyethylene socket and a cementless TPP. **c** Radiological status after 10 years. The position of the TPP is unchanged and shows no signs of loosening. The medial cortical bone shows increase in thickness

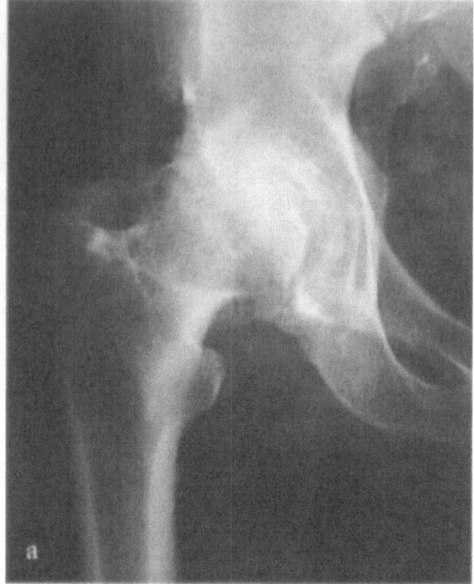

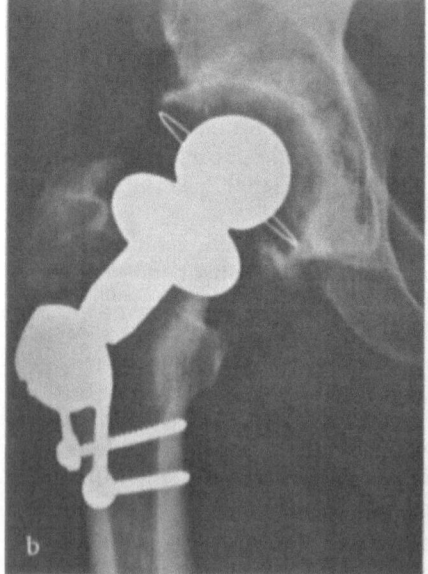

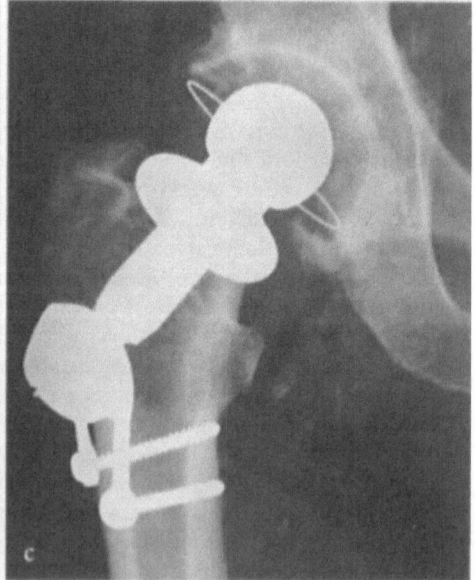

of aseptic loosening, 10-year survival was 86.2%. This considerable difference in 10-year survival is probably due to the relatively high proportion of cases of septic loosening. The results of the TPP are certainly comparable with those in a patient population of the same age group with conventional, cemented, total hip endoprostheses.

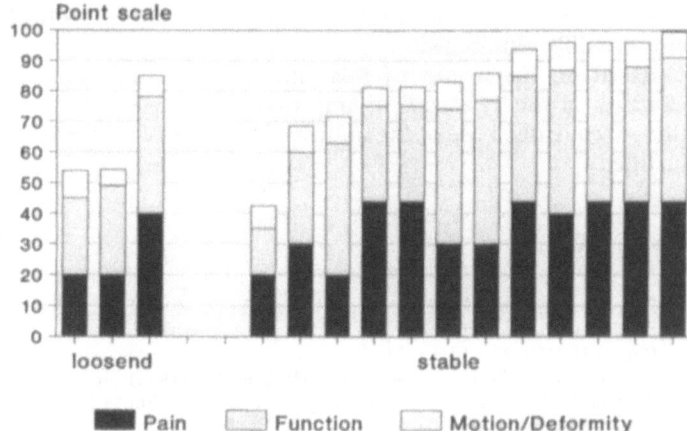

Fig. 7. Harris hip score for 15 nonrevised TPPs, classified according to the radiological finding "loose" or "not loose"

In contrast to femoral components with intramedullary fixation, the TPP concept has clear advantages:

- In the event of a revision operation the retreat to a femoral component with intramedullary fixation is very simple and almost comparable with a primary implantation.
- The concept excludes stress shielding of the proximal end of the femur; in no case was stress shielding observed. On the contrary, in about half of the nonrevised TPPs, a qualitative increase in the thickness of the medial cortical bone and the cortical structure was observed.
- There was no case of significant osteolysis in the proximal femur, even in the long term. Although only slight polyethylene wear was noticed in the acetabular socket, which may possibly be traced to the favourable properties of the rotational head, the thrust plate in fact appeared to seal off the proximal femur and thus provide protection against polyethylene wear debris and as a result, osteolysis.

Still unclear is the occasional phenomenon of a slight, gradual varization and a slight caudolateral shift of the TPP, even in pain-free patients. These cases showed an insignificant osteolysis line along the upper part of the mandrel of the TPP or a caudolateral displacement of the central bolt of some millimeters, and they may indicate a certain amount of deformation of the proximal femur in the long term.

The following design improvements as incorporated in the second and third generations of the TPP should improve the results over those reported above: Fractures of the lateral plate can certainly no longer occur, and with the through-hole in the mandrel the correct bolt length can be checked from the proximal end during the operation. The previous uncertainty as to the correct bolt length is thus eliminated. Changing the prosthesis material to a titanium alloy improves the osseointegration of the prosthesis, and the asymptomatic phenomenon of gradual varization and caudolateral shift of the prosthesis is also possibly eliminated.

Based on the results of this clinical pilot study and the conceptual advantages of the TPP with its improvement of possible weak points, the continued, controlled use of the improved TPP, presently in its third generation, is justified.

References

1. Huggler AH, Jacob HAC, Bereiter H, Haferkorn M, Ryf CH, Schenk R (1993) Long-term results with the uncemented thrust plate prosthesis (TPP). Acta Orthop Belg 59 [Suppl I]:215–223
2. Schreiber A, Jacob HAC, Suezawa Y, Huggler AH (1984) First results with the thrust plate Prosthesis. In: Morscher E (ed) The cementless fixation of hip endoprostheses. Springer, Berlin Heidelberg New York

CHAPTER 6

The Second-Generation Thrust Plate Prosthesis from 1988 to 1992

S. KERN

Introduction

Between September 1980 and April 1981, 20 thrust plate prostheses (TPPs) of the first series were implanted in a clinical trial at the Balgrist Orthopaedic University Clinic, Zurich. Based on the clinical experience obtained, subsequent small modifications were made to the implant. In May 1988 implantation of the further-developed and improved second generation of the TPP then began. In 1991 Kuhn presented the first comparison of the results with these two prostheses types[4]. All second-generation TPPs were implanted with the "Balgrist" hip socket. This is a tapered press-fit socket for cement-free implantation consisting of an outer expansion ring of pure titanium and an insert of polyethylene. Hauser reported in 1993 on the midterm results of this socket, which were found to be very good[1].

The TPP was used primarily for young patients, but the upper age limit was open, depending on various factors such as bone quality or osseous changes in the proximal femur.

Patient Population

Between 1988 and 1992 we implanted 31 TPPs of the second generation, all in combination with a cement-free Balgrist socket (for details, see Table 1). In the majority of cases (19/31) the indication for endoprosthetic treatment was idiopathic necrosis of the femoral head. The other causes were: 4 cases of dysplasia, 3 of arthrosis, and in 2 cases a steroid-induced necrosis of the femoral head. There was also one case each of epiphysiolysis, posttraumatic changes, and status following osteomyelitis of the proximal femur (Fig. 1). Two of the 31 hips had been previously operated on (intertrochanteric osteotomy). The left hip was affected in 17 cases and the right in 14. In 4 cases the prosthesis was implanted on both sides.

All patients were subjected to follow-up examinations using a standardized questionnaire after 3, 6, and 12 months and thereafter annually. Our prime interest in the follow-up examinations was the patient's subjective impression concerning pain and satisfaction.

Table 1. Second generation TPPs implanted (1988–1992; $n=31$)

	Men	Women
Number	28	3
Age range (years)	30–54	38–51
Median age (years; number)	42 (3/12)	45 (4/12)

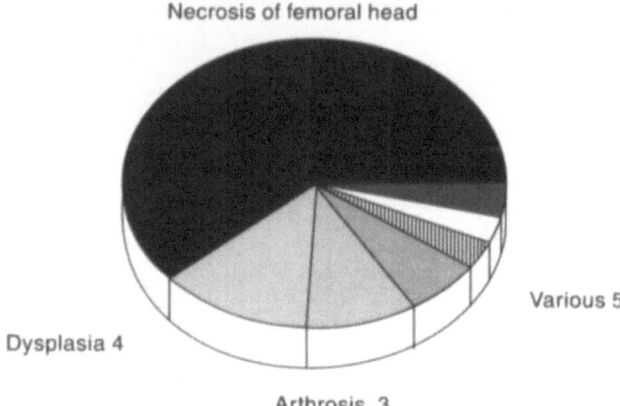

Necrosis of femoral head

Various 5

Dysplasia 4

Arthrosis 3

Fig. 1. Etiology of hip disorders treated with second generation TPP (n=31)

Results

More than two-thirds of the patients (22/31) rated the result of the operation positively (Figs. 2–4). Only two did not profit from the operation(Figs. 5 and 6). In terms of everyday activities 20 of the 31 reported little or no pain, 8 judged the pain to be quite tolerable, and 3 as strong. Of the 31 patients 25 felt they were not at all or were only slightly disabled, while 6 felt they were considerably restricted.

The following complications were encountered: With one patient an intraoperative pertrochanteric fracture of the femur occurred due to readjustment of the lateral plate that involved drilling additional holes in the cortex. This was treated by immobilization in a pelvis-leg cast. In another case the metal head which slipped off the end of the mandrel had to be replaced by one with a longer neck. In a further three cases a revision was necessary due to loosening of the central bolt. Up to now, a total of three TPPs of the second generation have had to be revised. The first case was aseptic loosening in the first year. The second was due to increasing varization of the TPP after full

Fig. 2a–c. Patient born 1958. **a** MRI sagittal section with practically complete femoral head necrosis. **b** TPP (*right*) with good seating on the medial femoral neck. **c** Implantation of a TPP (*left*) following full mobilization. Position more varus than the contralateral side, also with good medial seating

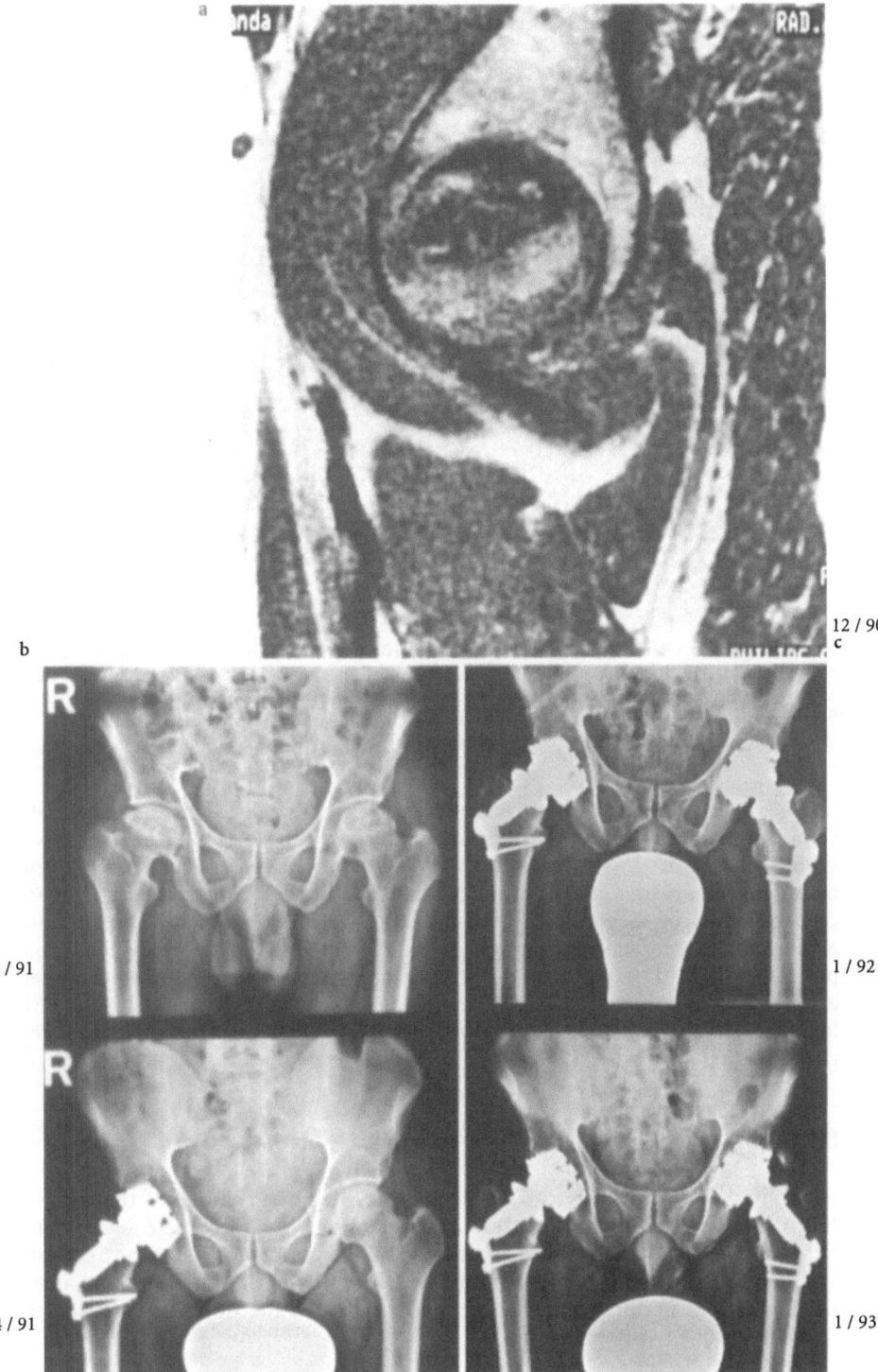

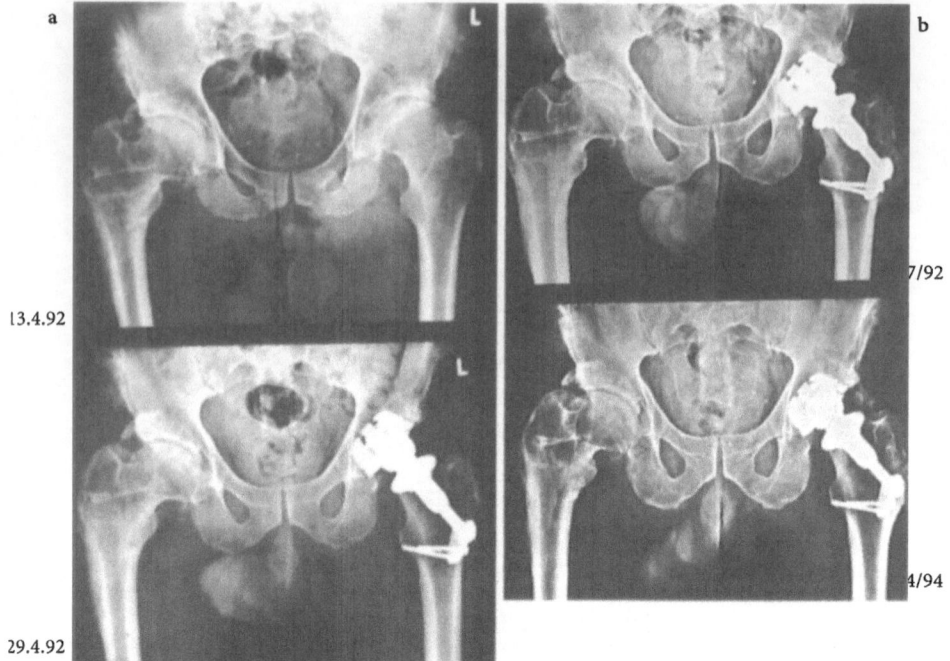

13.4.92

29.4.92

7/92

4/94

Fig. 3a,b. Patient born 1941. **a** Femoral head necrosis on both sides. *Right*, status following corrective intertrochanteric osteotomy; *left*, implantation of a TPP. Good seating of the thrust plate. **b** Radiological follow-up examination after 2 years. Appearance of periarticular ossifications, causing no difficulty subjectively or clinically. Clear remodelling of the medial femoral neck in the area of the thrust plate

loading was permitted. The mechanical stress was in fact so great that both screws in the lateral plate broke off. In this case the patient had previously undergone an intertrochanteric varization osteotomy which caused the TPP to be implanted in a distinctly varus position. The third TPP was revised because of complaints of discomfort in the area of the proximal femur. It did not exhibit any loosening intraoperatively and the osseous integration of the thrust plate appeared to be good (see Fig. 11, Chap. 2, this volume). However, even after replacement of this TPP by a conventional type of stem prosthesis (Alloclassic SL) there was no significant change in the subjective opinion of the patient.

Discussion

Basically a hip prosthesis can be fixed to the femur in either of three ways: intramedullar stem fixation, extracortical fixation using a conical socket, and fixation using a tension bolt or seating on the femoral neck stump [5]. Jacob and Huggler showed that the insertion of a hip prosthesis stem clearly changes the load transmission to the femur compared with the normal physiological

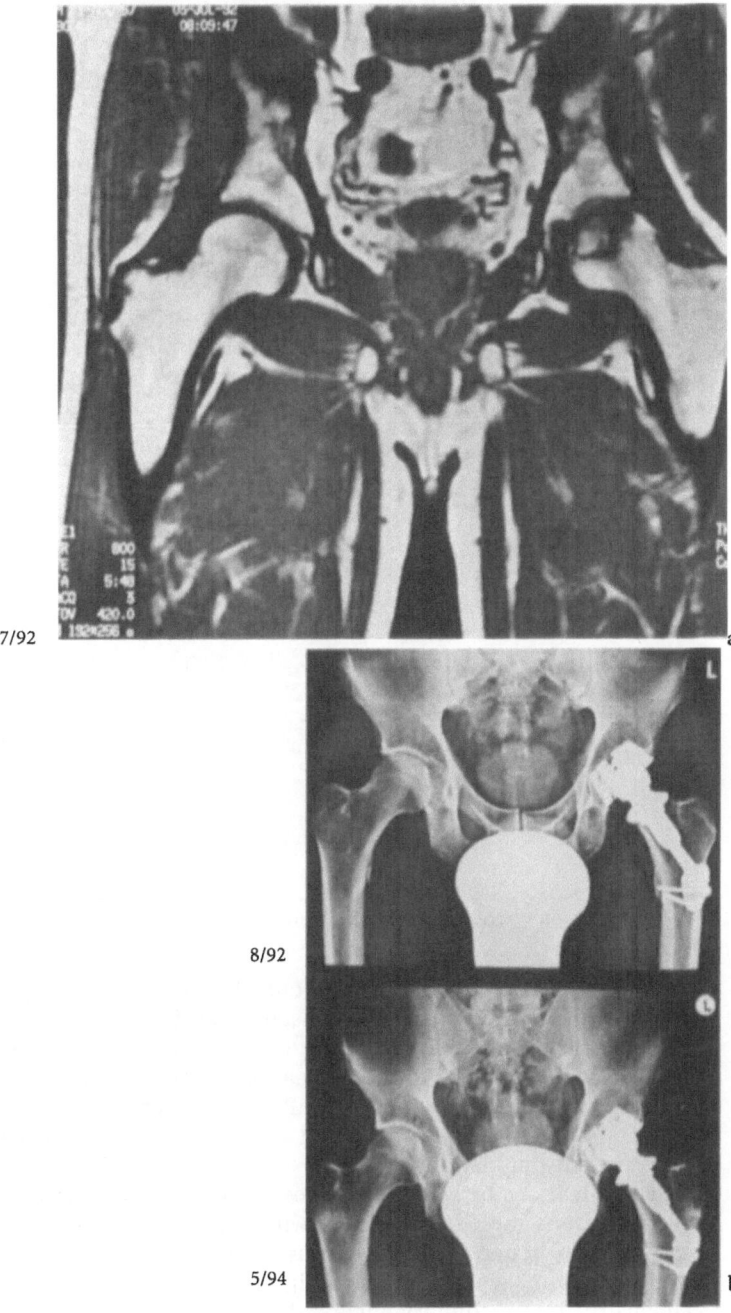

7/92   a

8/92

5/94   b

Fig. 4. Patient born 1957. **a** Femoral head necrosis shown by MRI. Large area of the head affected. Operation to save the joint no longer possible. **b** Follow-up examination 21 months after implantation of a TPP. Radiologically stable implant position

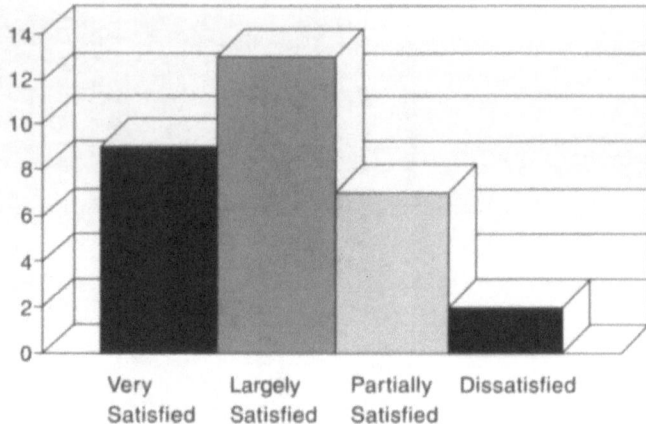

Fig. 5. Subjective assessment of second generation TPP ($n=31$)

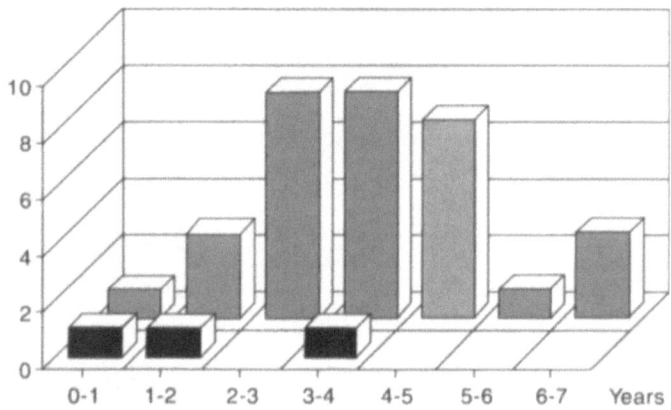

Fig. 6. Observation period for second generation TPP ($n=31$)

condition. A loading reduction of about 60% in the area of the femoral calcar is observed [3]. Based on these biomechanical findings, Huggler and Jacob in 1976 developed the TPP, with the objective of achieving a loading of the proximal femur as close to the normal physiological condition as possible [2]. The results of the first series of TPPs were so encouraging that in 1988 the implantation of the slightly modified second-generation TPP was started with a larger patient population.

Generally it can be said that the results with the TPP are good. However, for several reasons the clinical results with conventional hip prostheses may appear slightly better. This is because patients with TPPs are considerably younger than those with standard hip prostheses (average age of patients with cement-free intramedullary anchored prostheses is 54 years compared with 42 years in this study). Since younger patients are generally more active, they place more demands on the result of the operation and are therefore often less satisfied with it. Patients with the TPP are also a special population as regards etiology. Whereas arthrosis is present in over 50% of the cases in patients with a conventional cement-free total hip endoprostheses, this was so only in 10% of the patients with the TPP in our series. Idiopathic femoral head necrosis was diagnosed in 60% of the patients with the TPP, whereas this is the case in slightly over 10% with standard implants. (For further comments regarding femoral head necrosis and the TPP see Chap. 9, this volume.)

A revision rate of about 10% appears relatively high (3/31 TPPs have had to be revised to date). One case, however, concerns a stable implant, where the cause of pain remained unknown. The other two revision operations concern one case of early loosening in the first year and one in which the hip had been previously operated on (intertrochanteric varization osteotomy). In the latter the TPP could only be implanted in a varus position, and therefore upon commencement of full loading the force on the lateral plate was so great that the two cortical screws fractured. The conclusion to be drawn from this experience is that when there is a pronounced varus inclination of the femoral neck, the indication for a TPP must be examined carefully (see Chap. 1, this volume).

Each of the revision operations carried out showed us a further distinct advantage of the TPP: the implantation of a cement-free standard stem with intramedullary fixation could be carried out as if it were a primary implantation.

We can therefore summarize our experience with the second generation TPP as follows:

- To effect physiological load transfer from the implant onto the femoral neck stump, the TPP has a somewhat more complex form than conventional hip prostheses, which, however, should not present an experienced surgeon with any special problems during implantation.
- As there is no intramedullary fixation, implantation is possible even when there are certain malformations of the proximal femur, for example, following fracture or osteotomy. There is also an indication when, for instance, following osteomyelitis one does not want to enter the medullary canal.
- With the TPP the indication for implantation of a hip prosthesis can be extended to younger patients. Experience has shown that the later replacement of a TPP through a stem prosthesis with intramedullary fixation can be carried out easily, as if it were a primary implantation.

References

1. Hauser R, Jacob HAC, Kern S, Schreiber A (1993) Die Balgrist Hüftpfanne: eine 4–10-Jahres-Überlebenszeitanalyse von zementfreien Hüftpfannen. Z Orthop 131:585–593
2. Huggler AH, Jacob HAC (1984) The uncemented thrust plate prosthesis. In: Morscher E (ed) The cementless fixation of hip endoprostheses. Springer, Berlin Heidelberg New York, pp 125–129
3. Jacob HAC, Huggler AH (1978) Experimentelle Spannungsanalysen im menschlichen Oberschenkelknochen-Modell mit und ohne Prothese. Forschungsheft, Techn. Rundschau Sulzer, pp 73–83

4. Kuhn T (1991) Vergleichende klinische Studie der Druckscheiben-Hüftendoprothese: 40. Presented at the annual conference of the Vereinigung Nordwestdeutscher Orthopäden. ML Verlag
5. Ungethüm M, Blömer W (1987) Technologie der zementlosen Hüftendoprothetik. Orthopäde 16: 170–184

CHAPTER 7

Special Indications and Complications
with the Implantation of the Thrust Plate Prosthesis

U. SCHWARZENBACH

Introduction

Hip joint replacement has a particularly important place in orthopaedic implant surgery. The time span since the very first hip joint prostheses were implanted, the clinical results obtained up to now, and the biomechanical knowledge of the hip joint and femur far exceed the corresponding experience with any other artificial joint replacement. In the hip joint, with its clear anatomical and functional characteristics, endoprosthetic replacement is more favorable than in elbow or ankle joints due to the anatomy and the articular mechanics, which themselves place very complex demands on an implant.

Borderline indications and special situations raise questions of adaptability of the host bone to the demands of an implant, which differ from those imposed by normal physiological conditions. This chapter draws attention to the possibilities and limitations of the implantation of a thrust plate prosthesis (TPP) based on typical cases. In addition to the special indications, possible complications and the surgical means of eliminating them are also discussed.

Case Histories

Case No. 1

A woman aged 50 years. At the age of 20 this patient suffered a fracture of the proximal shaft of the femur, which at the time received conservative treatment. This resulted in a dislocatio ad axim at two levels. The medullary space remained obstructed at the level of the fracture. An increasingly painful coxarthrosis developed, which required surgical intervention. Figure 1a shows the situation before the operation. There was no means of implanting a conventional stem prosthesis, either cemented or cementless. Because of the small dimensions of the pelvis and the correspondingly small acetabulum, a suitable small prosthesis, model 40 S, would have been ideal, but at that time this size was not available. Figure 1b presents the result after implantation of a standard TPP, 1 year after surgery. Today, 3 years after the operation, the clinical result is functionally and radiologically excellent.

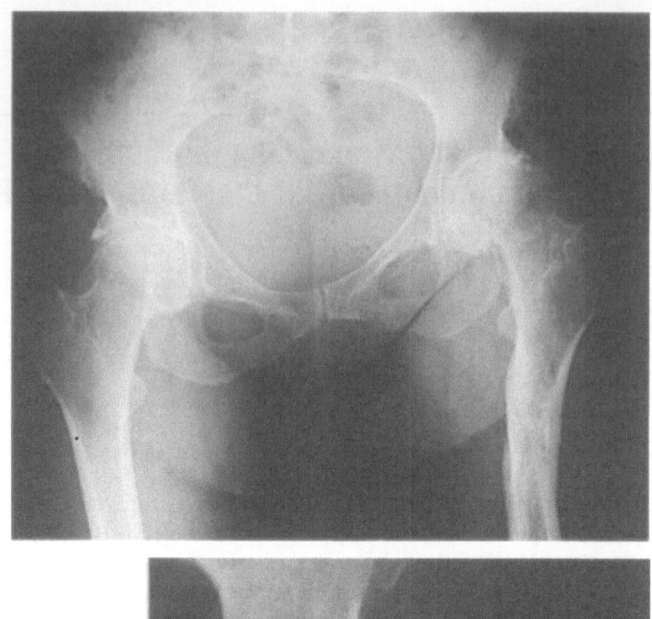

a

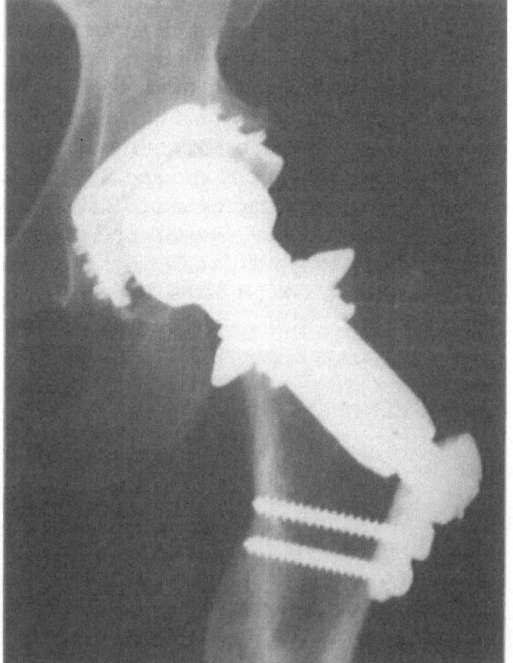

b

Fig. 1a,b. A 50-year old woman. **a** Painful osteoarthritis of the left hip. State after fracture with obliterated medullary cavity. **b** TPP 4 months after implantation

Case No. 2

A man aged 57 years (case of Dr. G. Meier, Chur, from the Cantonal Hospital, St. Gall). Osteopetrosis was diagnosed in this patient in 1990, at the time of a transpeduncular spondylodesis. The development of a painful left coxarthrosis indicated implantation of a total hip endoprosthesis (Fig. 2a). On the basis of experience gained at the time of the spondylodesis, it was decided that a standard prosthesis with intramedullary anchorage was hardly feasible because

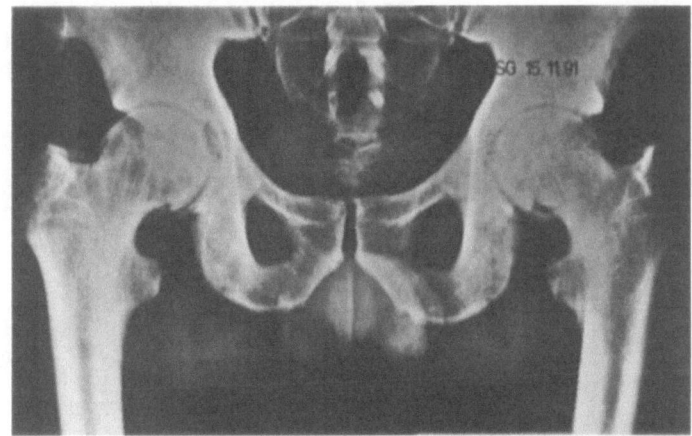

a

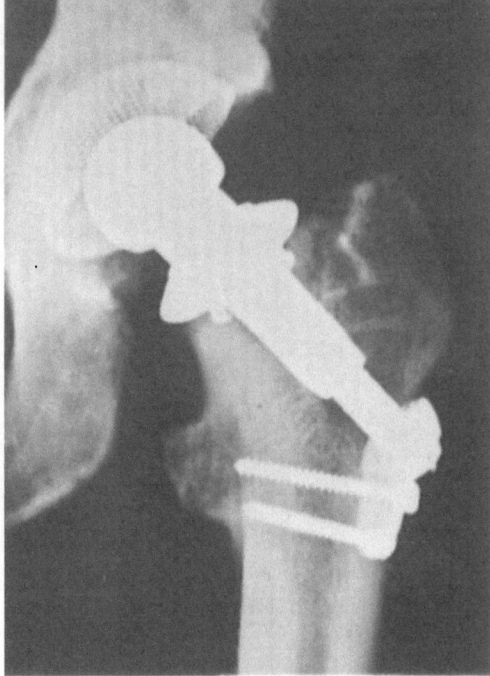

Fig. 2a,b. A 57-year-old man. **a** Osteo-petrosis with osteoarthritis of the left hip. **b** X-ray of the left hip 1 year after the implantation of a TPP

b

of the extremely hard bone. The use of a TPP was indicated. Even a freshly sharpened face milling cutter and with constant flushing allowed shortening of the neck of the femur by only 10 mm in 15 min. Three years after the operation the result is functionally and radiologically perfect (Fig. 2b).

Case No. 3

A man aged 38 years. Due to acute pain in the groin the patient underwent herniotomy at the age of 35, first on the right side and shortly afterwards on the left. With continuing pain, rapidly progressive necrosis of the head of the femur on both sides was discovered. Within a few months bilateral inter-

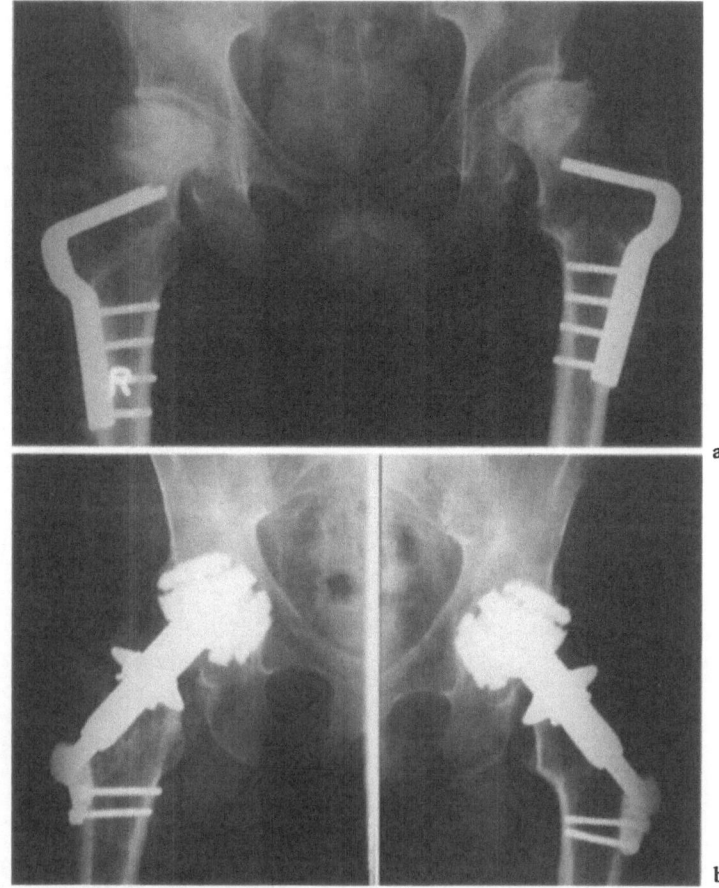

a

b

Fig. 3a,b. A 38-year-old man. **a** Bilateral femoral head necrosis. State after intertrochanteric osteotomies on both sides, which remained painful. **b** Two years six months after the insertion of a TPP bilaterally, the clinical result is excellent

trochanteric osteotomy was performed, and the necrotic material was drilled out. In spite of this the necrosis of the head of the femur continued to increase, and the joint surfaces broke down (Fig. 3a). The patient was almost unable to walk and had severe pain. He was then only 38 years old, and a TPP was therefore indicated; within half a year TPPs were implanted, first on the left side and then on the right. Two and a half years later the now 41-year-old butcher is again working normally. Functionally he is free from pain on both sides, and his hip mobility is unrestricted (Fig. 3b).

Especially in younger, active patients under the age of 60 years, stability and bone reactions of the osseous bed in the long term are of special interest. Decisive for the assessment of long-term results are undoubtedly the radiological parameters, which allow firm conclusions to be drawn for the indication of a TPP, to a far greater extent than subjective and clinical data.

With appropriate planning and a consistent, stepwise procedure, no complications are to be expected with the implantation of a TPP. Incorrect estimation of the bone consistency of its geometry can always result in a faulty implantation. This relates not only to the bone architecture of the central guide bore but also to the flat seating surface of the stump of the femoral neck on which the thrust plate rests. This aspect is discussed specifically in connection with case no. 4. Of the postoperative complications special mention should be

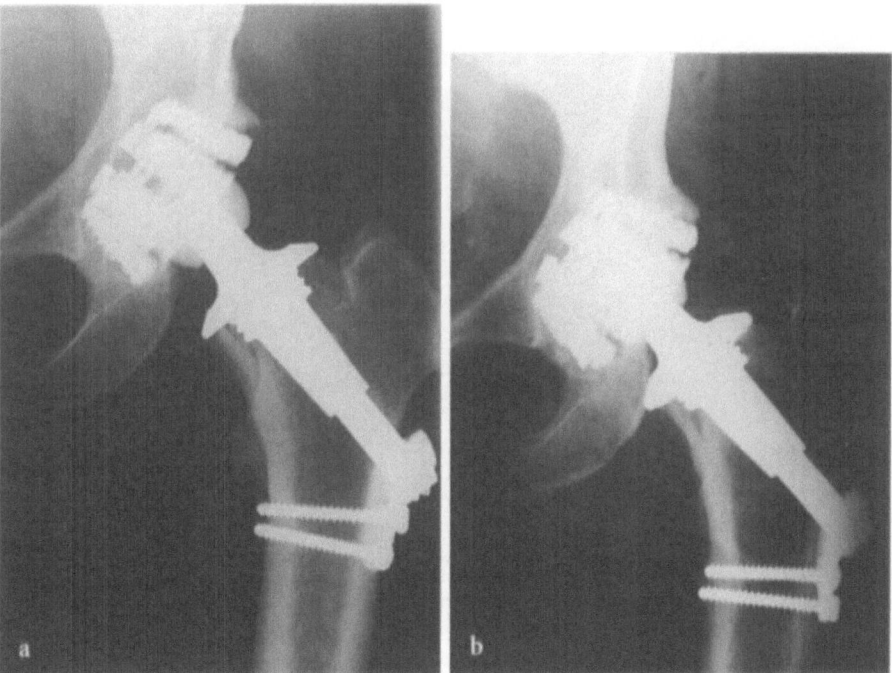

Fig. 4a,b. A 48-year-old woman. **a** The calcar was split when the TPP was inserted. **b** One year postoperatively the fracture has healed; the TPP remains stable

made of a fall injury that occurred in one case. The patient concerned, a woman, suffered a fracture of the femur on the first day after her discharge from hospital (case no. 5).

Case No. 4

A woman aged 48 years. A patient with a spastic hemisyndrome on the right side and bilateral coxarthrosis, which was somewhat more pronounced in the right hip, received a TPP implant on the left side. While driving in the thrust plate a fracture occurred in the region of the calcar femorale. Despite this the contact between the thrust plate and the stump of the femoral neck remained unimpaired. The implant was fixed stably only by tightening the central bolt sufficiently (Fig. 4a). After prolonged non-weight-bearing (4 weeks) mobility of the joint and consolidation of the fracture were unimpaired (Fig. 4b) (see Chap. 11, this volume).

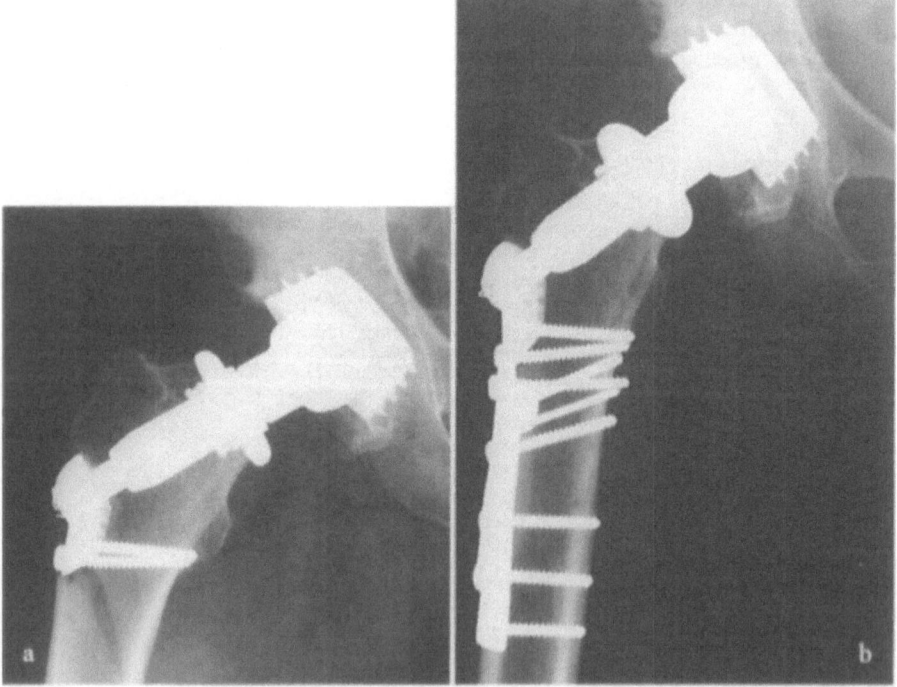

Fig. 5a,b. A 59-year-old woman. **a** At the lateral plate a short oblique traumatic fracture of the femur occurs. **b** Two weeks after the internal fixation of the fracture with two plates

Case No. 5

A woman aged 59 years. For many years this physically active patient had suffered from increasing pain in the right hip. With a wide femoral medullary space and a rather thin cortex layer, long-term stable anchorage of a conventional stem prosthesis was questionable. Therefore a TPP was indicated. Postoperative mobilization after implantation of the TPP was unproblematic, but unfortunately the patient had a fall at home a few days after leaving hospital, resulting in a fracture of the femur immediately below the lateral plate (Fig. 5a). By means of two T-plates placed one above the other and attached to the lateral plate it was possible to stabilize the fracture under compression. This led to rapid consolidation (Fig. 5b).

Discussion and Summary

The TPP has also proved its value in special indications. Particularly in cases in which the anchorage of a standard stem prosthesis could be problematic and the manufacture of a special prosthesis is not justified, the TPP can be used to advantage. This applies especially to younger, active patients. Complications such as perioperative fractures of the stump of the femoral neck or postoperative fractures of the femoral shaft resulting from a fall can also be stabilized by appropriate measures so that, in the event of a conventional stem-type prosthesis being required at some later date, no functional disadvantages for the patient result.

Although the examples mentioned here go back scarcely more than 3 years, the results as a whole can be described as positive. Questions regarding long-term results can be answered only by standardized radiological and clinical documentation, as only then can the adaptive reactions of bone in connection with the TPP be determined.

CHAPTER 8

Bone Remodelling of the Proximal Femur
After Implantation of a Thrust Plate Prosthesis

M. MENGE

Introduction

The major cause of long-term failure of hip endoprostheses is the biological behaviour of living bone. No foreign material is able to copy the physiological remodelling of the bone surrounding the prosthesis, so that interface problems become inevitable. Dispensing with bone cement causes problems with the partially unstable interface areas, which appear sooner and with more severity than with cemented prostheses that have a large area of stable fixation. The initial expectations for cementless stem endoprostheses were not met, and the problems were even aggravated. In comparison to patients with cemented implants [5], a relatively high proportion of patients with cementless fixation are dissatisfied with the early and mid-term results [2, 16, 18, 19, 21]. Mid-term results show that revision of cementless endoprostheses is required twice as often as in cemented arthroplasty [8, 10].

The essential mechanisms leading to aseptic loosening are also more evident with cementless implants than with cemented ones. Although radiology does not show osseointegration of the prosthesis, less radiopaque interface areas in radiographs indicate local areas with soft connective tissue and thus unsatisfactory anchorage. In contrast, secondary changes in the surrounding bone, such as changes in bone density, new trabecular orientation and changes in the cortical bone, signs of functional adaptation of the bone to the changed loading pattern, can be easily observed [6, 7, 24, 25, 27]. Bone remodelling, resulting from diaphysial wedging of a stiff prosthesis with distal load transfer, leads to proximal atrophy, formation of connective tissue and instability [23]; pain in the groin and upper thigh on loading and muscular instability with a Duchenne limp are understandable consequential results of this "partial loosening" [4, 18, 20, 22]. Figure 1 shows the functional remodelling of the bone as a result of the altered load transmission from the prosthesis stem to the diaphysial portion of the femur while bypassing the calcar femoris. Five years postoperatively, the 26-year-old patient is pain-free and satisfied, but limps and gets tired more rapidly on the right side. The radiograph shows the proximal part of the femur to be less radiopaque and atrophic, while only below the middle of the stem do trabecular structures provide evidence of osseointegration (grade III stress shielding according to Engh).

Apart from the functional adaptation of the osseous structures to the altered loading pattern, normal age-related bone remodelling and patient-specific

Fig. 1. A 26-year old man 5 years after implantation of a cementless titanium alloy prosthesis (type SKT, Orthoplant, Bremen). Whereas the proximal femur appears to have a cancellous bone structure and is atrophic, trabecular bone growth to the prosthesis stem in the distal half and cortical hypertrophy in the lower third are recognizable as functional adaptations to the stress shielding

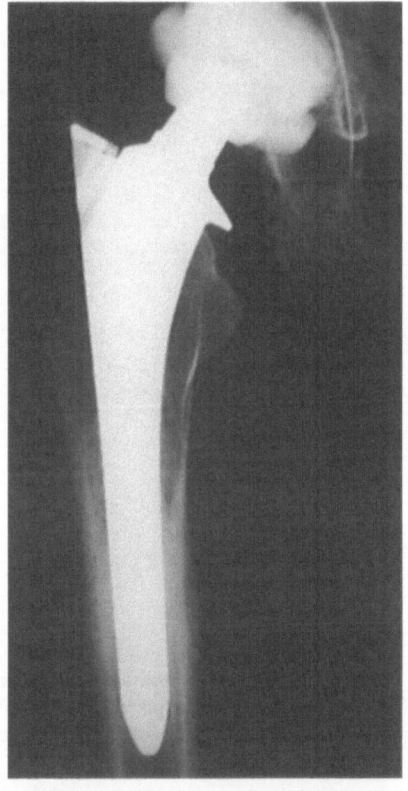

quality of the surrounding bone are important factors regarding the prognosis. In order to achieve the intended cancellous osseointegration, observation of the individual bone quality is very important. The micro-architecture of the cancellous bone undergoes change as a result of the aging process. Apart from an age-related reduction in the volume of cancellous bone, a sex-related difference can also be demonstrated. Above 50 years of age, women show significantly lower inter-trabecular linking compared to men of the same age [26]. This might explain the significantly higher frequency of femoral neck fractures in women. In addition, the more active bone remodelling in younger subjects [14, 15] with more rapid adaptation to altered loading patterns would explain the worse long-term results in this group of patients [10, 17].

From the osteological point of view, the direct loading of the resected surface with only metaphysial anchorage of the prosthesis would be advantageous, because stress shielding of the proximal femur would thus be avoided.

Due to the fact that, for an implant with only metaphysial fixation, sufficient stability for osseointegration cannot be achieved with certainty, even with optimum form-fit between the implant and the underlying bone [2, 23], initial stability must be provided by the use of screws or similar means. According to Huggler and Jacob, the thrust plate prosthesis (TPP; Fig. 2) meets these theoretical requirements. The thrust plate transfers the load to the cortical and

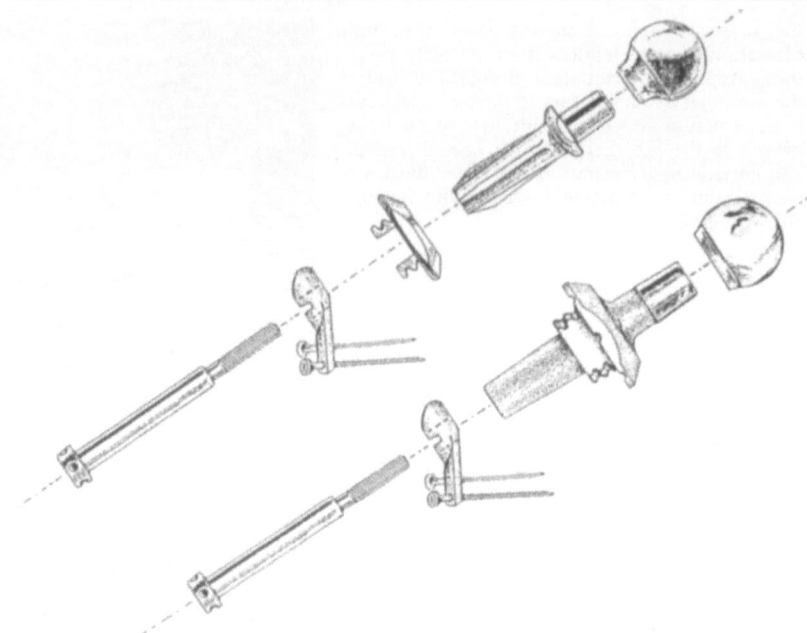

Fig. 2. The thrust plate prothesis (TPP), second (*top*) and third (*bottom*) series. In the new model, the thrust plate and the mandrel are combined into one prosthesis component, and the taper now permits the use of ceramic and metal ball heads

metaphyseal cancellous bone of the femoral stump. The central bolt with the lateral plate achieves pre-stressing, which guarantees stable primary fixation. In the long term, the thrust plate and the central bolt ensure exceptional rotational stability for a femoral implant by resting against the cortical bone. The TPP was first used in 1978 [11, 12], but until long-term results were available only small numbers were used [1, 9, 13].

Due to the biological reaction of the surrounding bone, as in any endoprosthesis, the concept cannot be validated by laboratory testing or biomechanical calculations alone, but on the basis of clinical results. This investigation therefore presents bone remodelling data resulting from implantation of the TPP.

Material and Methods

In the Ludwigshafen Orthopaedic Clinic, a total of 116 TPP were implanted from the beginning of 1991 until the middle of 1994 in 103 patients with an average age of 54.8 years (range, 28–78 years). Of these, 80 patients (69%) were able to be clinically and radiologically followed up; for a further 11 patients the family doctor has kept us informed of the patient's condition, and in eight

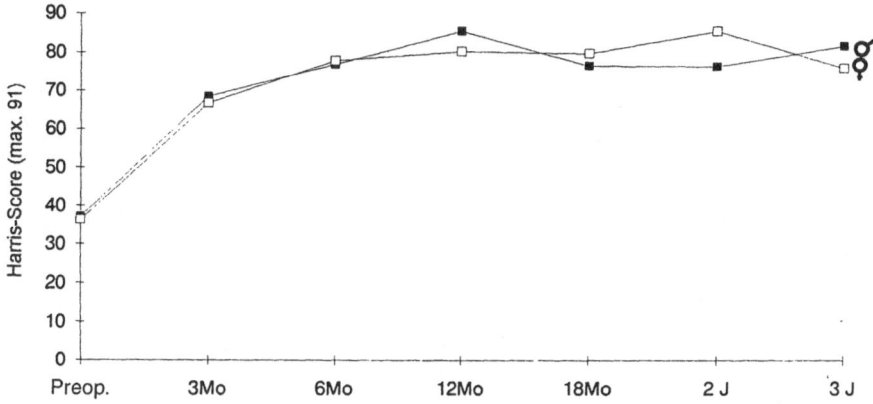

Fig. 3. Clinical results (pain and function scores) after implantation of the thrust plate prosthesis (TPP), according to gender (*black boxes*, males; *white boxes*, females). Values for 3 and 6 months, third series; longer-term results, second series

patients the condition has not yet been determined. The remaining 17 patients were not included in this study because the postoperative period is too short.

We used a grading questionnaire for the clinical follow-up examinations, giving ratings according to the usual scoring system. Because the patient ratings for "pain" and "mobility" are considered the most important, only these two quality attributes are shown in Fig. 3 using the simplified Harris Score (pain and function, maximum 91 points). The results for both sexes are the same, with a stable plateau reached after 1 year. It is noticeable, however, that although we found no gender-related differences in the clinical results in our patient population, the three cases of aseptic loosening (and one septic) occurred in women, which might possibly be due to the different quality of the cancellous bone (see above). Following varus tilting in one case of early loosening and in one previously inconspicuous case (Fig. 4), we have since tried to achieve a more valgus positioning of the prosthesis axis. This gave a mean increase in hip valgus of 5° in our total patient population. In rare individual cases, a femoral shaft-neck angle of nearly 150° was achieved; in these patients, the design-related adjustment limitations for the central bolt and the lateral plate led to technical difficulties during implantation.

The radiological follow-up examinations showed no significant change from the immediate postoperative condition in about half of the patients (52.7%). In one quarter of the cases (25.7%), however, we found characteristic functional reconstruction with remodelling of the compact structure of the calcar and the formation of trabecular structures towards the thrust plate. Apparently, the load in these patients is no longer transferred via the original cortical bone in the resection plane, but via new trabecular structures formed from the medial cortical bone. Figures 5 and 6 show such neo-trabeculae oriented towards the two anti-rotation pedicles on the underside of the thrust plate 1 and 2 years following implantation. In some cases, the solid cortical structure of the calcar

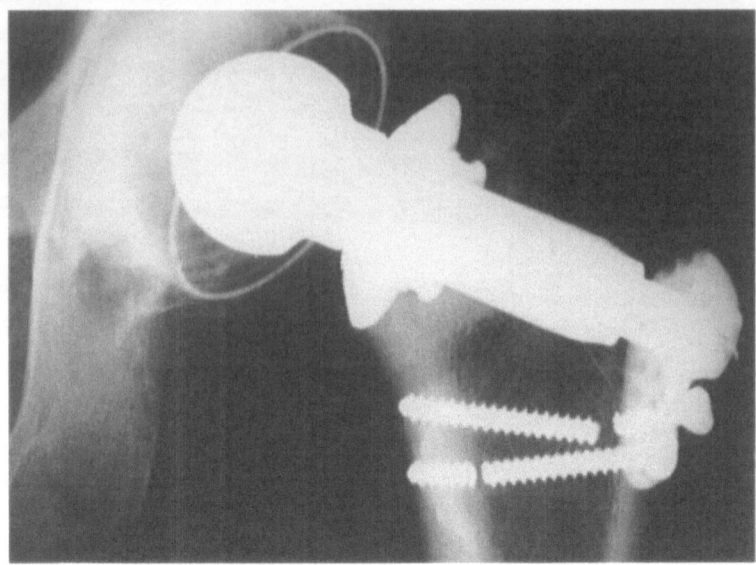

Fig. 4. Aseptic loosening in a 50-year old woman 18 months after implantation of a thrust plate prosthesis (TPP). The prosthesis has tipped to varus, and the lateral cortical screws have broken. The revision with a cemented stem prosthesis presented no problems

Fig. 5. A 62-year old woman 1 year postoperatively. The calcar has partially lost its compact structure, while new trabeculae are growing towards the medial "pedicle"

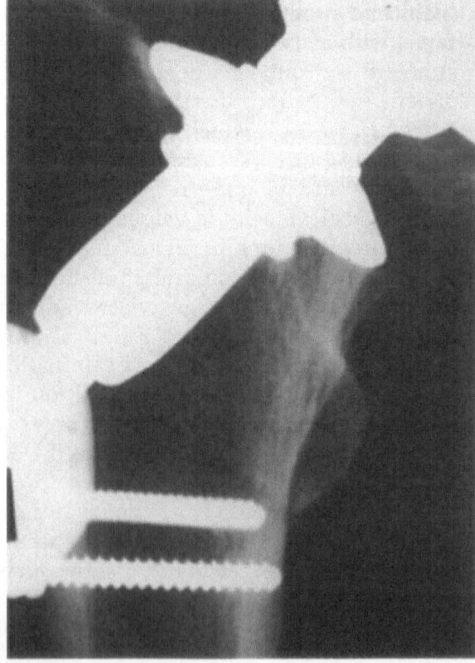

Fig. 6. A 58-year old woman 2 years after implantation of a thrust plate prosthesis (TPP). Trabecular remodelling with an outstanding clinical result

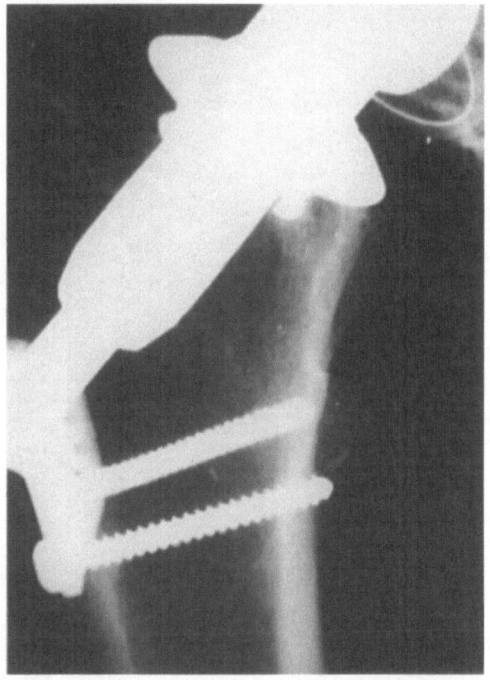

was transformed into trabecular bundles, and in others the cancellous bone support of the thrust plate was accompanied by the formation of connective tissue around the tapered section under the thrust plate or around the central bolt. Isolated formation of connective tissue was observed only infrequently. With two patients, follow-up showed formation of connective tissue around the tapered section under the thrust plate together with varus movement of the implant. It is possible that this movement will terminate in aseptic loosening.

The design of the lateral plate and the central bolt was based on a femoral shaft-neck angle of 125°. In two cases with varus tilting, fracture of the lateral cortical screws occurred. In three women (Fig. 4), we therefore tried intra-operatively to achieve a valgus positioning of the implant. An extreme valgus position is not without problems, however; in six patients with a femoral shaft-neck angle of over 140° (mean, 143.4°), we observed increasing atrophy under the medial portion of the thrust plate with corresponding sclerosis of the lateral seating area (Fig. 7). However, there were two patients with coxa vara and consequently a prosthesis in varus position (about 115°) right from the start which has remained stable up to now. Due to the variety of possibilities for interpretation, aseptic loosening cannot be explained solely on grounds of positioning.

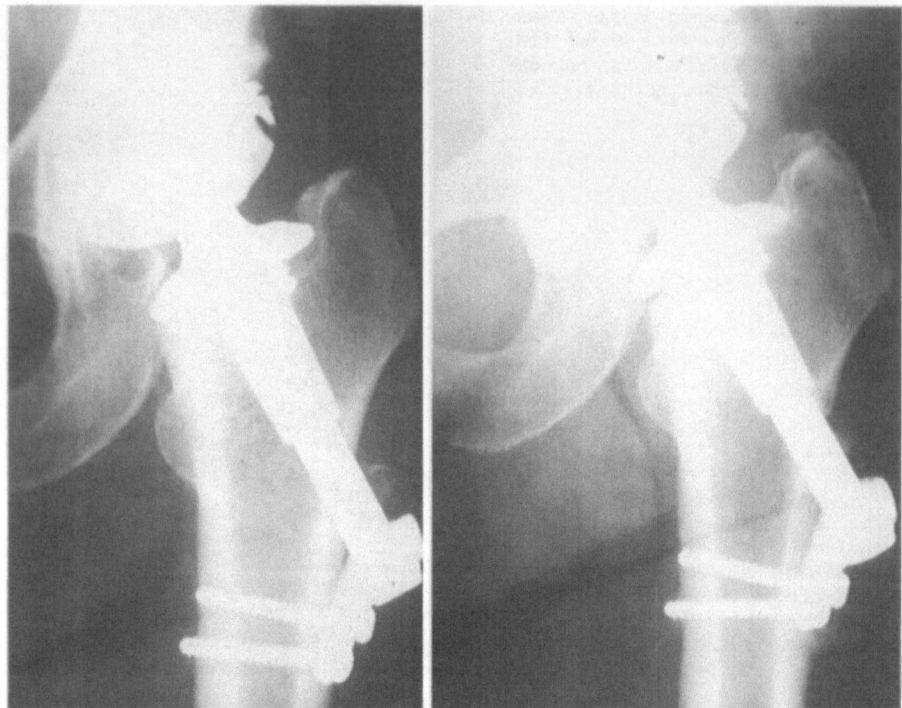

Fig. 7. A 53-year old woman immediately following operation (*left*) and 6 months later (*right*). The valgus position of 148° led to remodelling with partial resorption of the calcar with secondary medial formation of a gap and with zones of sclerosis below the lateral thrust plate. No clinical problems

Discussion

Almost one quarter of the patients in our clinic who receive hip implants are under 60 years of age (22.6%). While the earlier cemented prostheses proved to be sufficiently reliable for older patients, arthroplasty for patients with a longer life expectancy remained problematic. Revision methods to date, using even longer implant stems, remained unconvincing, because bone loss close to the joint and insufficient proximal medullary cavity quality due to failure of the first attempt worsen the prognosis for the second prosthesis. The TPP, a metaphysial femoral prosthesis, appears to offer a solution to this dilemma. Primary treatment restricted to the metaphysial zone is potentially able to greatly postpone the use of a standard prosthesis. The TPP results in our patient population confirm at least the short and mid-term satisfactory method of treatment. This is true even though some patients still have slight pain, particularly in the lateral plate area. Despite the remaining symptoms, nine patients decided to have the other side treated with a TPP as well; the extent of the remaining discomfort thus appears to be tolerable.

The radiologically detectable functional adaptation reactions in just over one quarter of the cases indicate the remodelling that occurs in younger patients as a result of the altered loading pattern. In these cases, the TPP principle of proximal loading leads to functional adaptation with the development of a new trabecular load transfer system in place of the former calcar femoris. The aseptic loosening rate of 2.6% over the observation period was clearly higher than that for conventional cemented prostheses in a much older population (1.7%), but still below the revision rate (3.9%) for conventional cementless ones [10]. Aseptic loosening in our patient population has so far occurred only in women (50, 51 and 56 years old); prognosis might therefore be affected by gender-specific osteopenia. Whether daily activities of the patients will equal or exceed that known for standard procedures is still open, but, in contrast to stem prostheses, the ability to carry out revisions is technically unproblematic. From the point of view of surgical technique and duration, replacement with a cemented or cementless standard prosthesis does not differ from a primary operation.

In my own experience (admittedly only nearly 3 years), the TPP has proved to be at least as good for younger patients as previous cemented prostheses over this period. At this point in time, the TPP may be regarded as a valid alternative for younger patients with stable osseous structures.

References

1. Bereiter H, Jacob HAC, Huggler AH (1986) Die klinischen Erfahrungen mit der Druckscheibenprothese. Med Orthop Tech 1: 21–23
2. Brown IW, Ring PA (1985) Osteolytic changes in the upper femoral shaft following porous-coated hip replacement. JBJS 67-B: 218–221
3. Burke DW, O'Connor DO et al (1991) Micromotion of cemented and uncemented femoral components. JBJS 73-B: 33–37
4. Campbell ACL, Rorabeck CH, Bourne RB (1990) Thigh pain and cementless total hip arthroplasty: a clinical and radiological correlation. JBJS 72-B: 539
5. Dall DM, Learmouth ID, Salomon MI (1988) Charnley low friction arthroplasty: the yardstick. JBJS 70-B: 499
6. Engh CA, Bobyn JD (1985) Biological fixation in total hip arthroplasty. Slack, Thorofare, NJ
7. Engh CA, Bobyn JD, Glassman AH (1987) Porous-coated hip replacement. JBJS 69-B: 45–55
8. Harris WH, Maloney WJ, Barrack RJ et al (1993) Cement vs cementless for the femoral component. Modern cement wins. Orthop Transact 17: 68
9. Hauser R (1994) Die Druckscheibenprothese – eine Pilotstudie von 20 Fällen über 10 Jahre. Vortrag auf der 42. Jahrestagung der Vereinigung Süddeutscher Orthopäden, 30 Apr 1994
10. Havelin LI, Espehaug B, Vollset SE, Engesaeter LB (1994) Early failures among 14,009 cemented and 1,326 uncemented prostheses for primary coxarthrosis. Acta Orthop Scand 65: 1–6
11. Huggler AH, Jacob HAC (1983) Die zementlose Druckscheibenhüftendoprothese. In: Morscher E (ed) Die zementlose Fixation von Hüftprothesen. Springer, Berlin Heidelberg New York, pp 128–133
12. Huggler AH, Jacob HAC (1984) The uncemented thrust plate hip prosthesis. In: Morscher E (ed) The cementless fixation of hip endoprosthesis. Springer, Berlin Heidelberg New York, pp 125–129
13. Huggler AH, Seemann PS (1987) Die Druckscheibenprothese im siebten Jahr ihrer klinischen Anwendung. In: Draenert K, Rütt A (eds) Beiträge zur Implantatverankerung. Hist Morph Bewegungsapp 3: 171–184

14. Kummer B (1989) Normales Skelettwachstum unter anatomischen und funktionellen Gesichtspunkten. In: Willert H-G, Heuck FHW (eds) Neuere Ergebnisse der Osteologie. Springer, Berlin Heidelberg New York, pp 31–39
15. Küsswetter W, Gabriel E, Stuhler T, Töpfer L (1983) Spongiosierungsvorgänge im femoralen Knochenlager konventionell implantierter Hüftprothesen. In: Morscher E (ed) Die zementlose Fixation von Hüftprothesen. Springer, Berlin Heidelberg New York, pp 16–19
16. Maaz B, Menge M, Maaz M (1985) Komplikationen nach Implantation des zementfreien BMO-Stufenschaftes (Frialit-System). Z Orthop 123: 649–650
17. Malchau H, Herberts P et al (1993) Prognose der totalen Hüftarthroplastik. 61st annual meeting of the American Academy of Orthopedic Surgeons, San Francisco
18. Menge M (1985) Klinische Erfahrungen mit dem System Zweymüller-Endler: Analyse der Folgebeschwerden. In: Maaz B, Menge M (ed) Aktuelle Probleme der zementfreien Hüftendoprothetik. Thieme, Stuttgart, pp 44–50
19. Menge M (1988) Derzeitiger Stand und mittelfristige Ergebnisse von Neuentwicklungen bei zementierten Schaftendoprothesen. In: Maaz B, Gierse H (eds) Aktueller Stand der zementfreien Hüftendoprothetik. Thieme, Stuttgart, pp 43–55
20. Menge M (1991) Preßfit und Zementmantel – ein Widerspruch? In: Gierse H, Maaz B (eds) Die Hüftendoprothetik. ecomed, Landsberg, Germany, pp 105–114
21. Menge M (1995) Die metaphysäre Prothesenverankerung: ein neues Prinzip für die Femurprothese. Orthop Prax 31: 94–102
22. Menge M, Maaz B, Lisiak B (1985) Komplikationen nach Implantation des zementfreien Titanschaftes nach Zweymüller. Z Orthop 123: 648–649
23. Nunn D, Freeman MAR, Tanner KE et al (1989) Torsional stability of the femoral component of hip arthroplasty. JBJS 71-B: 452–455
24. Oh I, Harris WH (1978) Proximal strain distribution in the loaded femur. JBJS 60-A: 75–85
25. Perren SM (1983) Induktion der Knochenresorption bei der Prothesenlockerung. In: Morscher E (ed) Die zementlose Fixation von Hüftprothesen. Springer, Berlin Heidelberg New York, pp 38–40
26. Pompesius-Kempa M, Hahn M et al (1989) Neue Untersuchungen zur Mikroarchitektur der Spongiosa bei Osteopathien im Vergleich zu altersbedingten Veränderungen. In: Willert H-G, Heuck FHW (eds) Neuere Ergebnisse der Osteologie. Springer, Berlin Heidelberg New York, pp 206–210
27. Wolff J (1892) Das Gesetz der Transformation der Knochen. Hirschwald, Berlin

CHAPTER 9

The Thrust Plate Prosthesis in Osteological Disorders

W. Rüther, B. Fink, T. Schneider, and E. Kornely

Introduction

Not only the anatomical circumstances and/or the pathomechanical conditions at the proximal end of the femur are of special significance for the long-term behaviour of the thrust plate prosthesis (TPP), but also inherent properties of the bone itself and its reactions to the altered load pattern. The increasing density of bone beneath the thrust plate over time can be radiologically detected [3, 4, 15, 16]. Where primary or secondary disease of the bone is present, the question of "bone quality" in the areas of the femoral metaphysis and diaphysis also needs to be addressed. In these cases it cannot be taken for granted that the periprosthetic bone can withstand the altered mechanical loads or that it is capable of adjusting sufficiently to the changed load pattern. Particular attention must be paid to this aspect in prostheses that are metaphysially anchored.

In the Orthopaedic Clinic of the University of Düsseldorf, the TPP has been used since February 1992. We report on 59 prostheses that were implanted in patients under 50 years of age. The indications were various forms of arthrosis, arthritis and osteonecrosis (Table 1). Special attention was paid to osteonecrosis when using the TPP with metaphysial fixation, because it cannot be simply assumed that the metaphysial and diaphysial bone is not included in the underlying disease process.

Periprosthetic Densitometry

Periprosthetic bone density measurement using dual-energy X-ray absorptiometry (DEXA) is available as a means of achieving earlier or more detailed visualization or even quantification of the reactions of the bone to the TPP and also of the changes in the distribution of bone density than is possible with radiography. Bone density measurement in the proximal femur is already an established method for the diagnosis of osteoporosis. Periprosthetic densitometry permits measurement of significant changes in bone density with a satisfactory degree of accuracy [5, 20]. Various evaluation methods have been proposed for femoral stem prostheses and have been reviewed in a relatively short series of investigations to date [18, 31]. No such analyses are yet available for the TPP. In the following, preliminary data are presented and periprosthetic measurement areas are proposed.

Table 1. Descriptive statistics of the indications for operations using a thrust plate prosthesis (TPP) from February 1992 to June 1994

Indication	Operation (*n*)
Arthrosis	24
Arthritis	6
Osteonecrosis	29
Induced by alcohol	8
Following kidney transplantation	7
Following leukaemia therapy	3
With lupus arthritis	1
Other cortisone medication	2
Not classified	8
Total	59

Immediately following the endoprosthetic replacement of the hip joint with a TPP, the density distribution of the proximal femur is seen to be very similar to that before implantation and/or to that on the non-operated contralateral side (Fig. 1). The bone of the proximal femur generally remodels over time. In Fig. 2, an increase in bone density can be seen caudal below the thrust plate 1.5 years after implantation, while the density actually appears to decrease in the area of the mandrel. The qualitative changes are less apparent in Fig. 3; however, when using reproducible measuring zones, a clear increase in bone mass is detectable over the course of 2 years. Using segmented measurements, the cranial zones, i.e. those areas immediately beneath the thrust plate, prove to be the ones with the highest density increase.

In two patients in which varus movement of the TPP was observed, densitometry showed quite different activity. In the case of a 40-year-old alcoholic patient (Fig. 4), pronounced osteosclerosis below the thrust plate developed within 2.5 years. A slight varus movement of the prosthesis was detected in radiographs at the same time. The patient is completely symptom-free, shows an excellent clinical result and has resumed his previous job as a driver. The

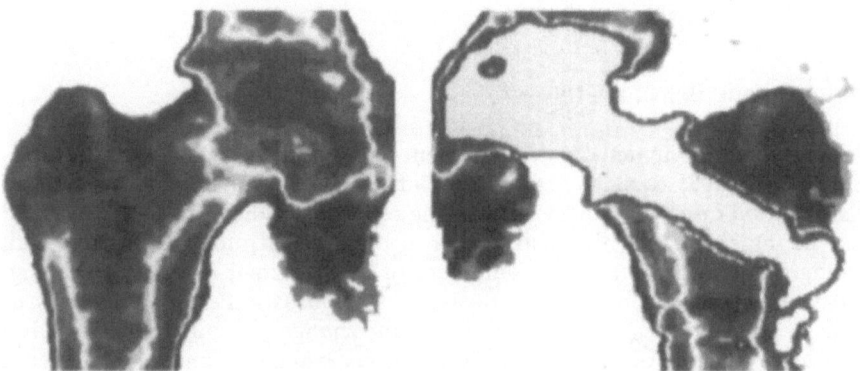

Fig. 1. Simultaneous comparison of bone density left and right, showing no significant differences

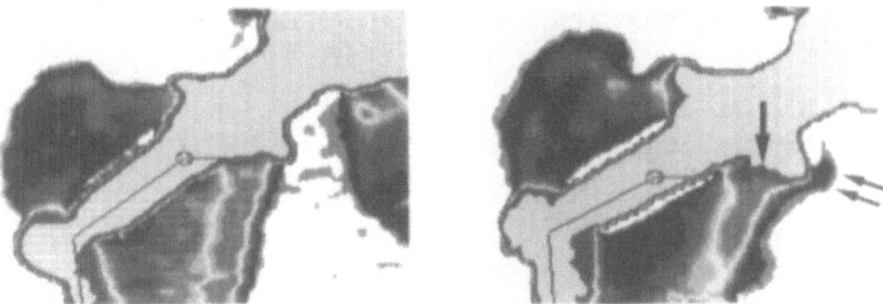

Fig. 2. Densitometric results in periods of 1.5 years (indication was femoral head necrosis following therapy of acute lymphatic leukemia). The bone density immediately caudal to the thrust plate is increasing (*arrow*), while the density appears to decrease in the area of the prosthesis shaft and the trochanter major. A curved osseous spur has formed at the caudal edge of the thrust plate (*double arrow*)

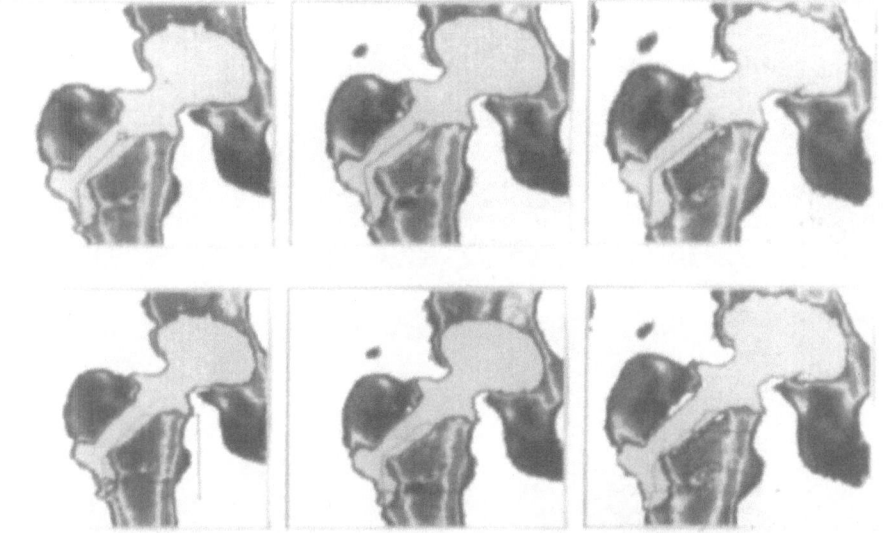

a

b

Fig. 3a,b. Indication was dysplasia coxarthrosis. The densitometric picture shows that only minor remodelling has occurred over a period of 2 years. Clear changes are indicated by the density measurements. **a** The quantification is done using reproducible measuring zones and shows an increase in density over 2 years. **b** Using segmented measuring zones, the cranial areas, i.e. those immediately beneath the thrust plate, prove to be those with the greatest density increase

second patient (Fig. 5) was a 27-year-old man with renal osteopathy. Multi-articular osteonecrosis appeared following kidney transplantation. The radiograph shows a slight varus movement of the TPP 1.75 years following its implantation. Not even the beginnings of an increase in bone density can be detected radiologically or using densitometry. The clinical result is excellent.

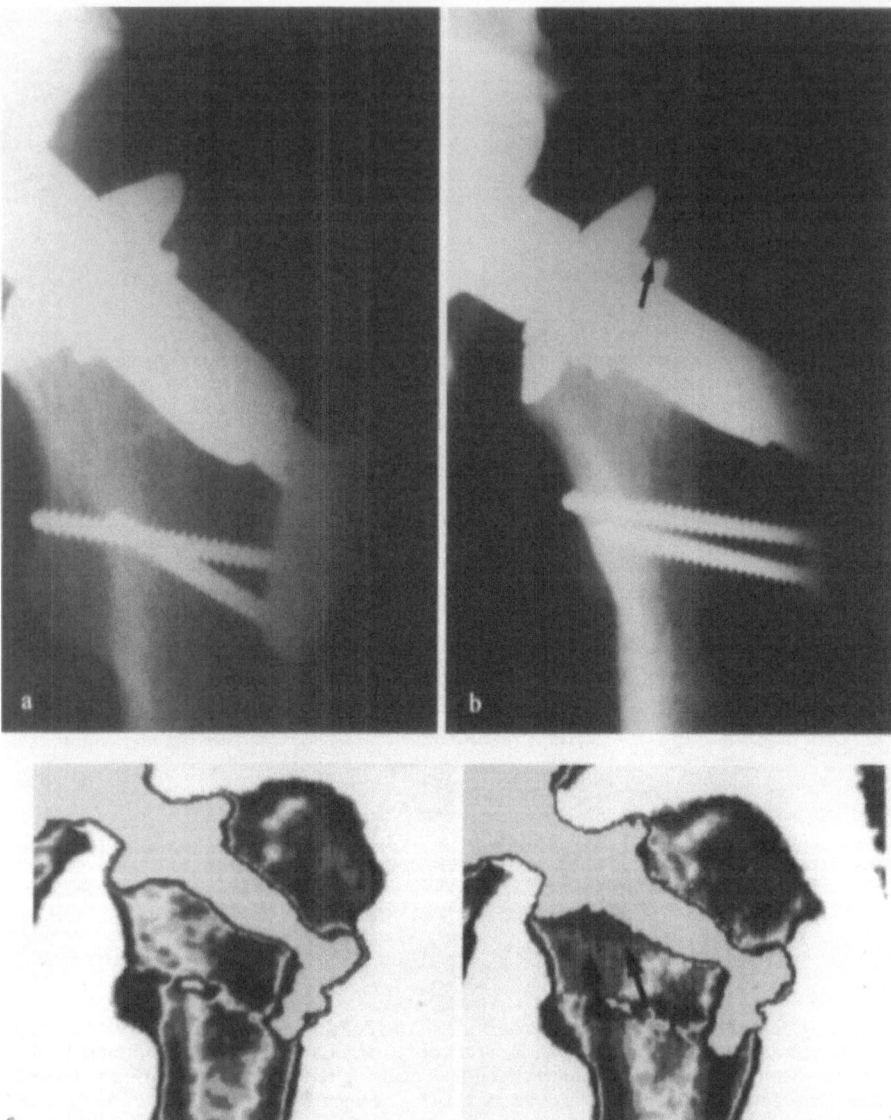

Fig. 4a–d. A 40-year-old man, alcoholic, with femoral head necrosis. Radiographs taken **a** 1 month and **b** 2.5 years following endoprosthetic replacement; a slight varus movement of the prosthesis (*arrow*) and a clear densification in the osseous structure beneath the thrust plate can be seen. **c** Using densitometry, the increase in the bone density (*arrow*) can be clearly followed. **d** The preoperative magnetic resonance imaging (MRI) picture (here in the T2-weighted picture) shows the extension of the necrosis well into the femoral neck (*arrow*)

Fig. 4d

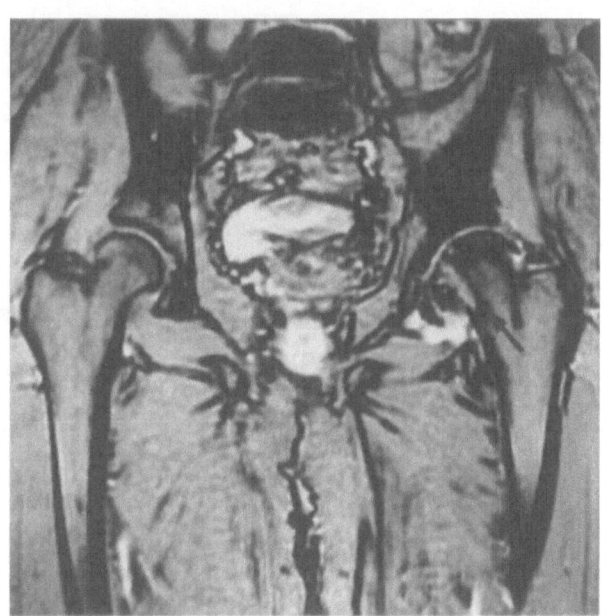

Due to the limited experience with periprosthetic bone density measurements with the TPP, no analysis of the causes of the different processes has yet been possible. Sintering and loosening of the implant also still remain a mystery. The measurements are, however, reproducible with sufficient accuracy, and the method therefore appears very promising.

The Thrust Plate Prosthesis with Femoral Head Necrosis

In 29 patients in the investigated population, the TPP was implanted due to osteonecrosis. The maximum of 2.5 years' observation time to date is short. Within this period, change of position of the femoral implant, i.e. in varus, was observed in four patients; two of these patients were men who had had kidney transplants (Fig. 5), another man suffered from alcoholism (Fig. 4), and one woman had idiopathic femoral head necrosis. There is no clear answer to the question of whether these developments are related to the basic disease or whether these are phenomena associated with the TPP. It is significant, however, that similar developments were never observed in any of the 30 patients in which the TPP was implanted due to arthrosis or arthritis. Furthermore, it is remarkable that, in all four patients, osteonecrosis in the area of the acetabular socket was evidenced using magnetic resonance imaging (MRI) and in some cases histologically [11]. It can at least be concluded that the osteonecrosis in these cases was not restricted to the femoral head alone.

There are generally higher loosening rates following endoprosthetic replacement of the hip joint due to non-traumatic femoral head necrosis than

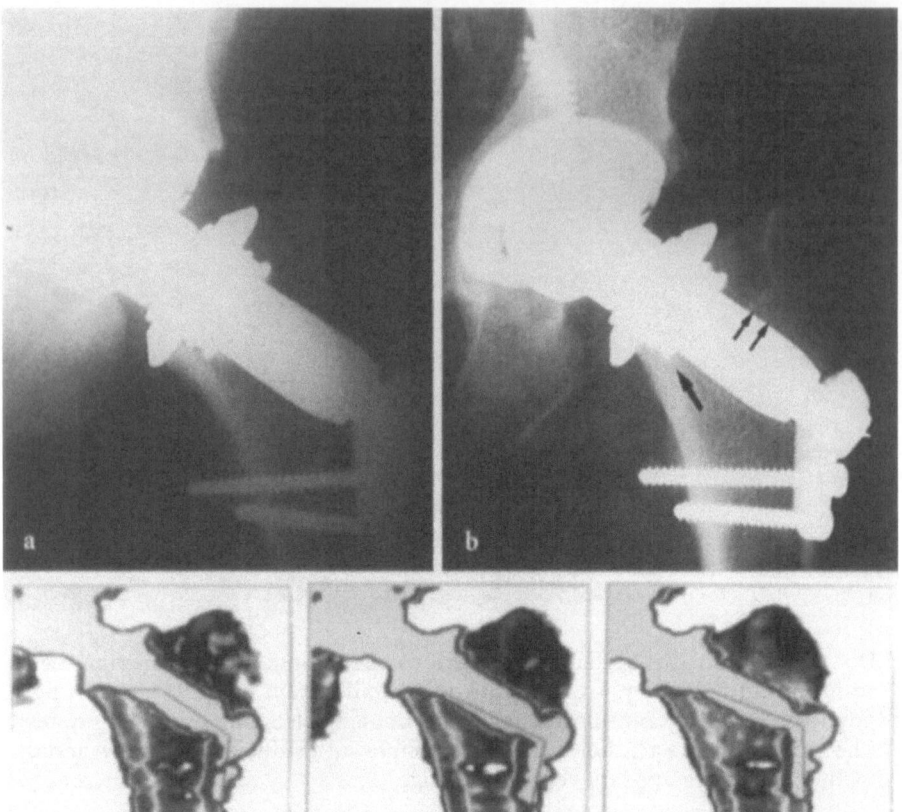

Fig. 5a–c. A 27-year-old patient following kidney transplantation with multiarticular osteo-necrosis. The radiograph reveals no changes in the osseous structure **a** 1 month and **b** 1.75 years following the operation. The implant has moved slightly to varus (*arrow*), and an osseous double contour can be seen on the cranial side of the prosthesis shaft (*double arrow*). **c** The densitometric picture shows no significant change of the structural density. The clinical result is very good

when due to coxarthrosis or traumatic femoral head necrosis. This applies not only for cup arthroplasty [27], but also for hemi-prostheses [29] and for cemented and cementless total endoprostheses [28, 30]. Thus, 7.6 years after implantation of cemented total prostheses following non-traumatic femoral head necrosis, Cornell et al. found an average loosening rate of 37%; Saito et al. [28] found 28% after 7 years, and Schneider et al. [30] 77% after 9.1 years. Clarke et al. and Hanker et al. observed prosthesis loosening rates of 59% and 56%, respectively, after 5.5 years in cases of femoral head necrosis caused by sickle cell anaemia.

Most authors attribute the higher loosening rate of endoprostheses in mostly younger patients with non-traumatic femoral head necrosis to increased physical activity and corresponding higher mechanical loading of the prosthesis. The higher osteometabolism of younger subjects may also be a significant factor.

Independently of this, factors must be taken into account which are directly the cause of or are indirectly associated with femoral head necrosis; at the same time, due to reduction of the metaphysial "bone quality", they should be considered the cause of early prosthesis loosening [10, 22, 28–30]. Moreover, the following must be considered in various disorders: reduction of the local osteoblast activity (cortisone and alcohol inter alia), accompanying metabolic osteopathy (e.g. renal osteodystrophy), extension of the zone of necrosis into the metaphysis and diaphysis (e.g. renal osteodystrophy, sickle cell anaemia or as a sequela of leukaemia therapy) and disturbance in the perfusion of the bone as a systemic disease (isolated necroses beyond the intracapital necrosis zone, early adiposity of the marrow).

Reduction of Osteoblast Activity

It must be accepted that cortisone medication and abuse of alcohol lead to osteoporosis. Additionally, there is significant reduction in osteoblast activity. Arlot et al. [2] found a marked reduction in osteoblast activity in pelvic crest samples from patients with non-traumatic femoral head necrosis. Osteoporosis and reduced osteoblast activity can cause defects in the healing of micro-fractures [29]. The osseointegration of the prosthesis, i.e. the trabecular re-modelling of the proximal end of the femur, can then be slowed down or even completely arrested.

Metabolic Osteopathy

This alteration becomes pronounced when basic metabolic disease is additionally present, as is the case, for example, with renal osteodystrophy. The chronic insufficiency of the kidneys leads to various changes in the bone, which can be traced essentially to disturbances in vitamin D metabolism and to hyperparathyroidism. Hyperparathyroidism itself is the result of insufficient renal phosphate excretion, which leads to hyperphosphataemia, and the result of a renal disturbance in the hydroxylation of vitamin D, which initiates hypocalcemia. Histologically, the bone shows fibro-osteoclasia and osteomalacia in differing ratios. The picture is overlaid with the effects of medication, e.g. cortisone and aluminium [1, 13]. Finally, secondary amyloidosis can impair the bone [9].

Hip-joint problems in kidney patients are therefore not only the result of chronic kidney insufficiency, but also the result of kidney transplantation with medication effects, e.g. from cortisone. Many problems are the sequelae of other problems. Osteonecrosis is apparently not only the result of cortisone use, but can appear as nephrogenic osteopathy [10, 23].

Finally, MRI of patients with kidney insufficiency frequently shows changes in the bone marrow which cannot be classified with certainty, but which are

Fig. 6. A 50-year-old patient following kidney transplantation. In the magnetic resonance imaging (MRI) picture, diffuse, inhomogeneous, irregularly shaped reductions in signal intensity can be seen in the fatty marrow of the femur, possibly as a result of fibro-osteoclasia

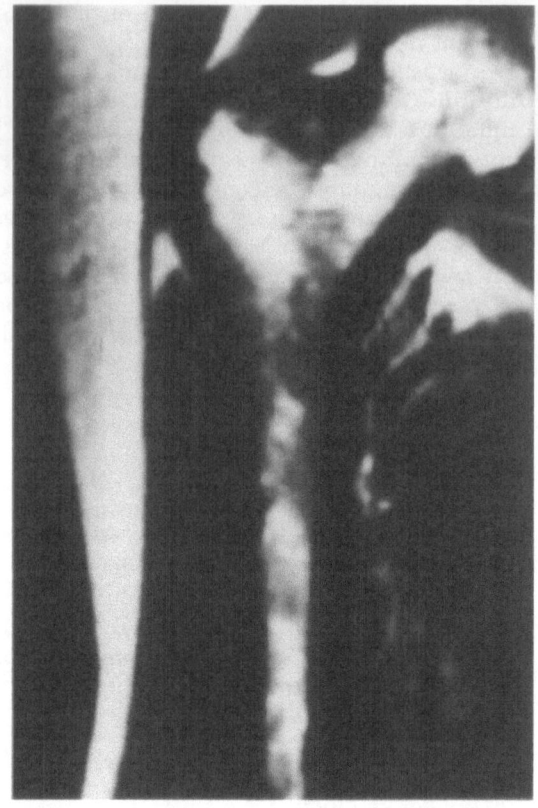

possibly the result of fibro-osteoclasia in the context of hyperparathyroidism. This appears as diffuse, inhomogeneous, irregularly shaped reductions in signal intensity in the fatty marrow of the femoral shaft, which can affect the whole femur (Fig. 6). Meßler et al. [21] found these conspicuous areas in 62% of the patients investigated with kidney insufficiency.

The complex disturbance of osteometabolism alters the mechanical properties of the bone. Osteosynthesis is disturbed [32]. A slowing down of the bone remodelling processes to accommodate the changed load pattern following endoprosthetic hip joint replacement must also be expected.

In the literature concerning endoprosthetic hip joint replacement in patients with renal osteodystrophy, there is little or no reference to the very different individual initial conditions of the bone. As a rule, a hip endoprosthesis in a patient with renal osteodystrophy is indicated for femoral head necrosis following kidney transplantation. Most authors describe the loosening rate in the mid-term as significantly increased [6, 7, 8, 19, 24–26]. High rates of early complications (20% [6]) and of late infection (13%; [19]) are reported. However, Romero et al. [26] achieved such good long-term results that they saw no impairment of prosthesis fixation due to renal osteopathy and steroid-induced osteoporosis and recommended cementless hip prostheses for patients with kidney transplants as well. In a similar manner, Frassica et al. [12] prefer a short-stemmed cementless femoral implant for transplant patients.

Among our seven patients with kidney transplants, there were two in which the TPP showed early varus movement, diagnosed after 3 and 18 months, respectively. There was distinct renal osteopathy in both cases. One patient received continuous cortisone medication for rejection therapy (Fig. 5). In the second patient, there was continued tertiary hyperparathyroidism despite parathyroidectomy.

Local Extension of Osteonecrosis

The local extension of femoral head necrosis varies considerably. Primary and secondary implant stability is unimpaired when a cemented or cementless stem prosthesis is used, even where the necrotic activity reaches as far as the metaphysis of the femoral neck. However, the TPP relies explicitly on vital, metabolically active bone tissue in the area of the femoral neck. One should therefore be fully acquainted with the extent of necrotic activity before implantation. MRI is best suited for this.

Figure 5c shows femoral head necrosis, extending a good distance into the femoral neck, as a result of alcoholic abuse. The osteotomy was performed just below the necrosis. Particularly after cortisone therapy for leukaemia, the necrotic areas can conquer large parts of the endostal cavity (Fig. 7). In these patients, the use of a TPP should not be considered.

Fink et al. [11] have recently pointed out that in the course of femoral head necrosis the acetabular region may also be osteonecrotic. Such developments have been observed principally in patients with chronic polyarthritis [14, 17]. Although the condition of the acetabular region is of no direct consequence for the use of a TPP, acetabular necroses are still to be regarded as an indication that necrosis is not limited to the intracapital area, but that the whole periarticular bone might be affected to a greater or lesser degree. In the four observed cases of change in position of the TPP, osteonecrosis of the acetabulum was also present.

Disturbance in the Perfusion of the Proximal Femur

In eight of 11 patients with femoral head necrosis, Saito et al. [28] found additional isolated necroses in the femoral head and neck, beyond the intracapital area of osteonecrosis, that extended into the area of the calcar femoris and the intertrochanteric region. Early stem loosening occurred in seven of these eight patients, preceded by resorption of the calcar. The authors conclude that there is a close correlation between isolated femoral neck and calcar necrotic areas and calcar resorption, with early prosthesis loosening. Accordingly, with femoral head necrosis, not only is the intracapital region affected, but also the femoral neck, possibly even the whole metaphysis and diaphysis, as a systemic intra-osseous arteriolar disease.

Fig. 7. A 48-year-old patient following kidney transplantation with femoral head necrosis. The endostal extension of the necroses is well into the femoral diaphysis (here in a T1-weighted picture)

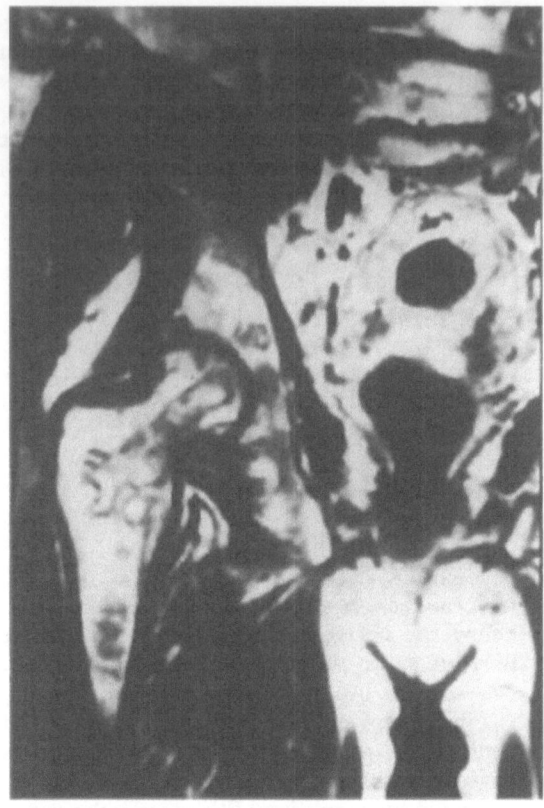

Mitchell et al. [22] described early adiposity of the femoral bone marrow, identified by MRI, in patients under 50 years of age with femoral head necrosis. The replacement of the haematopoietic bone marrow in this region by fatty marrow has been suggested to be the result of a reduction in perfusion, which in the case of femoral head necrosis extends over the whole proximal end of the femur.

Summary

For its long-term success, the TPP requires osseous integration and calls for some adaptation of the bone to the slightly changed biomechanical loading of the proximal femur. When metabolic bone disease is present, it cannot be simply assumed that the remodelling processes will take place to the necessary extent. In apparently locally isolated configurations of femoral head necrosis, there are many indications that, in addition to the intracapital area, alterations in other parts of the proximal femoral bone have taken place where the biological quality of the affected bone reduces its suitability for the TPP.

The periprosthetic measurement of bone density using the DEXA method appears suitable for the observation of the remodelling of bone surrounding the prosthesis. Where osteonecrosis is present, MRI may be considered before implanting the TPP, in order to obtain definitive information on the spread of the necrosis. For patients with femoral head necrosis and renal osteodystrophy, there does not appear a priori any additional risk of early prosthesis loosening; however, the experience to date does not permit evaluation of the risk factors with certainty.

References

1. Almond MK, Kvan JT, Evans E, Cunningham J (1994) Loss of regional bone mineral density in the first 12 month following renal transplantation. Nephron 66: 52–57
2. Arlot ME, Bonjean M, Chavassieux PM et al (1983) Bone histology in adults with aseptic necrosis: Histomorphometric evaluation of iliac biopsies in seventy-seven patients. J Bone Joint Surg 65A: 1319–1327
3. Bereiter H, Jacob HAC, Huggler AH (1986) Die klinischen Erfahrungen mit der Druck-scheibenprothese. Med Orthop Techn 21–23
4. Bereiter H, Huggler AH, Jacob HAC, Seemann P (1991) The thrust plate prosthesis. A new concept in hip prosthesis design eight years of clinical experience. Orthop Rel Sci 2: 191–202
5. Bobyn JD, Mortimer ES, Glassmann AH, Engh CA, Miller JE, Brocks CE (1992) Producing and avoiding stress shielding: laboratory and clinical observations of non-cemented total hip replacements. Clin Orthop 274: 79–86
6. Bradford DS, James PC, Simmons RS, Najarian US (1983) Total hip arthroplasty in renal transplant recipients. Clin Orthop 181: 107–114
7. Chemell SJ, Schwartz CM, Giaccdhino JL, Ing TS (1983) Total hip replacement in patients with renal transplants. Arch Surg 113: 489–495
8. Devlin VJ, Einhorn TA, Gordon SL, Alvarez EV, Butt KM (1988) Total hip arthroplasty after renal transplantation. Long term follow up study and assessment of metabolic bone status. J Arthroplasty 3: 205–213
9. Düreke TB (1991) Beta-2-microglobulin amyloidosis and renal bone disease. Miner Electrolyte Metab 17: 261–272
10. Fink B, Rüther W, Busch T, Schneider T (1993) Multiple aseptische Knochennekrose bei chronischer Hämodialyse. Osteologie 2: 228–232
11. Fink B, Rüther W, Schneider T, Assheuer J (1994) Aseptische Knochennekrosen des Acetabulum. In: Neuere Ergebnisse in der Osteologie. Springer, Berlin Heidelberg New York
12. Frassica FJ, Kavanagh BF, Morrey BF (1991) Avascular necrosis. In: Morrey BF (ed) Joint replacement arthroplasty. Churchill Livingstone, New York, pp 765–777
13. Goodman WG, Duarte MEL (1991) Aluminium: effects on bone and role in the pathogenesis of renal osteodystrophy. Miner Electrolyte Metab 17: 221–232
14. Hipp E, Glas K (1987) Idiopathische Hüftkopfnekrose. In: Witt AN, Rettig H, Schlegel KF (eds) Orthopädie in Klinik und Praxis. Thieme, Stuttgart, pp 2.65–2.107
15. Huggler AH, Jacob HAC (1984) The uncemented thrust plate hip prosthesis. In: Morscher E (ed) The cementless fixation of hip endoprostheses. Springer, Berlin Heidelberg New York, pp 125–129
16. Huggler AH, Seemann P-S (1987) Die Druckscheibenprothese im siebten Jahr ihrer klinischen Anwendung. Hist Morph Bewegungsapp 3: 171–184
17. Kida Y, Katom Y, Yamada H, Tsuji H (1993) Extensive osteonecrosis of the acetabulum in a patient who had rheumatoid arthritis. J Bone Joint Surg 73A: 930–931
18. Kirath BJ, Heiner JP, McBeath AA, Wilson MA (1992) Determination of bone mineral density by dual x-ray absorptiometry in patients with uncemented total hip arthroplasty. J Orthop Res 10: 836–844
19. Lo NN, Tan JS, Tan SK, Vathsala A (1992) Results of total hip replacement in renal transplant recipients. Ann Acad Med Singapore 21: 694–698

20. McCarthy CK, Steinberg GG, Argen M, Leahey D, Wyman E, Baran DT (1991) Quantifying bone loss from the proximal femur after total hip arthroplasty. J Bone Joint Surg 73B: 774–778
21. Meßler H, Fink B, Klehr U, Steudel A (1989) Der Einfluß unterschiedlicher Parameter auf die Entstehung der aseptischen Hüftkopfnekrose bei Nierentransplantierten unter besonderer Berücksichtigung des NMR. In: Willert HG, Heuck FHW (eds) Neuere Ergebnisse in der Osteologie. Springer, Berlin Heidelberg New York, p 510
22. Mitchell DG, Steinberg ME, Dalinka MK, Rao VM, Fallon M, Kressel HY (1989) Magnetic resonance imaging of the ischemic hip. Clin Orthop 244: 60–77
23. Nishiyama K, Okinaga A (1993) Osteonecrosis after renal transplantation in children. Clin Orthop 295: 168–171
24. Radford PJ, Doran R, Greatorex A, Rushton N (1989) Total hip replacement in the renal transplant recipient. J Bone Joint Surg 71B: 456–459
25. Rombouts JJ, Pirson Y, Squifflet JP, Vincent A, de-Nayer P et al (1992) Aseptic necrosis of the femoral head following renal transplantation: assessment of a 25 year experience. Acta Orthop Belg 58: 373–387
26. Romero J, Schreiber A, Binswanger U, Müller H (1991) Totalendoprothesenarthroplastik nach Nierenallotransplantation. In: Stuhler T (ed) Hüftkopfnekrose. Springer, Berlin Heidelberg New York, pp 729–739
27. Safran MR, Amstutz HC (1991) Nontraumatic osteonecrosis. In: Amstutz HC (ed) Hip arthroplasty. Churchill Livingstone, New York, pp 639–675
28. Saito S, Saito M, Nishina T, Ohzono K, Ono K (1989) Long term results of total hip arthroplasty for osteonecrosis of the femoral head. Clin Orthop 244: 198–207
29. Salvati EA, Cornell CN (1988) Long-term follow-up of total hip replacement in patients with vascular necrosis. Mosby, St Louis, pp 67–73 (American Academy of Orthopaedic Surgeons Instructional Course Lectures XXXVII)
30. Schneider E, Ahrendt J, Niethard FU, Bläsius K (1989) Save the joint or replace it. Z Orthop 127: 163–168
31. Trevisan C, Bigoni M, Cherubini R, Steiger P, Randelli G, Ortolani S (1993) Dual x-ray absorptiometry for the evaluation of bone density from the proximal femur after total hip arthroplasty: analysis protocols and reproducibility. Calcif Tissue 53: 158–161
32. Zichner L (1988) Therapie von Knochen- und Gelenkveränderungen bei renaler Osteodystrophie im Erwachsenenalter. Orthopäde 17: 440–447

CHAPTER 10

The Limits of Indications for the Thrust Plate Prosthesis

G. GRUBER and H. STÜRZ

Primary and secondary coxarthroses are the main indication for the thrust plate prosthesis (TPP) with cement-free implantation (Figs. 1 and 2). The target group for the implantation of a TPP comprises mainly younger patients. The age limit does not depend, of course, on the actual age of the patient but rather on the biological age, his/her wishes for mobility and activity, and the social environment. For patients under 50 years of age the decision to operate requires a strict diagnosis, as with every joint replacement operation. Due to the potential for reduced osseointegration on account of disease, the TPP should not be used as a standard prosthesis in patients with pronounced osteoporosis or compensated kidney insufficiency or in patients of any age on dialysis. Similar considerations also apply in the case of femoral head necrosis, as the biological quality of the femoral neck cannot be clearly established.

Given a normal anatomical frame, the normal geometry of the hip joint can as a rule be maintained using a TPP. The prosthesis permits the reconstruction of a femoral neck angle of between 125° and 135° with antetorsion between 10° and 15° and a normal femoral neck length. However, even with normal femoral neck angles there are limitations in the use of the prosthesis, namely in cases where the femoral neck is short, and where the diameter of the femoral neck is below a critical minimum limit so that the central mandrel under the thrust plate no longer fits into the femoral neck. The seating surface of the mandrel of the smallest model is 24 mm high and 18 or 14 mm wide in the largest and narrowest sections, respectively. The inside diameter of femoral neck which is to receive the prosthesis must not be smaller. Where the femoral neck diameter is at the lower limit, forced implantation can lead to fissure or fracture of the femoral neck. Coxa vara, with a typically short femoral neck, or residual hip joint dysplasia with pathologically increased antetorsion, can present technical operating problems during implantation. The relatively short femoral neck prevents the application of sufficient compression on the thrust plate, so that preference should be given to conventional endoprosthetic treatment in these special cases (see Figs. 5, 6, 8).

Apart from femoral neck diameter, femoral neck length also limits the use of the prosthesis in its present dimensions. When using the shortest bolt, the smallest distance between the lateral plate and the thrust plate is 35.1 mm for the size 40 thrust plate, and 40.1 mm for the size 44 thrust plate. When using a head with standard neck length and 28 mm diameter, the necessary minimum length of the femoral neck stump is 78.1 mm, measured from the inner edge of

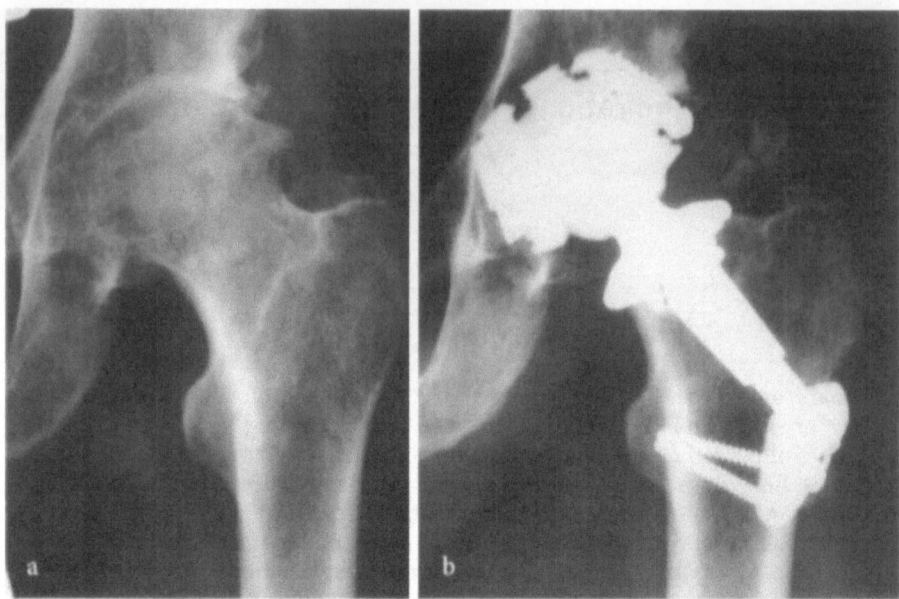

Figs. 1a,b. Pre- and postoperative radiological status of a 51-year-old man with coxarthrosis and head necrosis on the left side

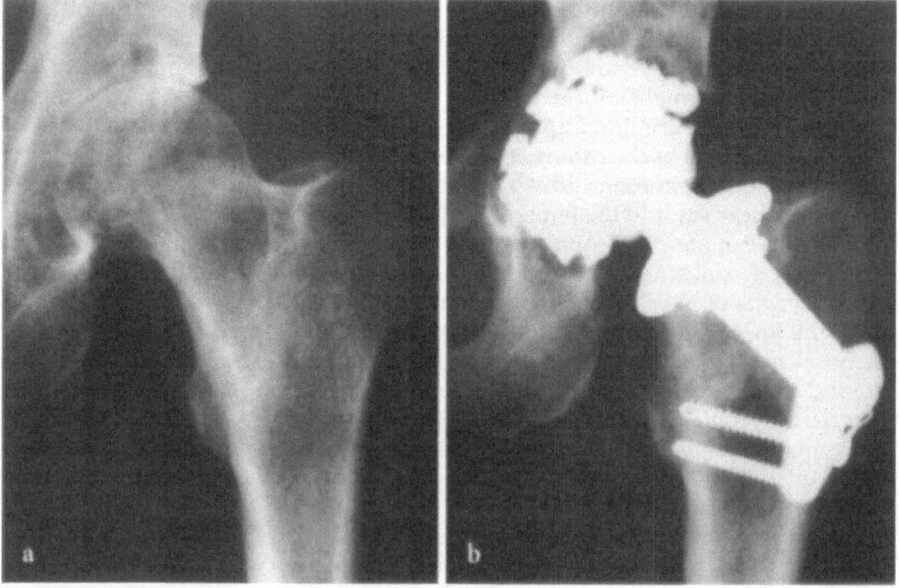

Figs. 2a,b. Pre- and postoperative radiological status of a 62-year-old woman with coxarthrosis on the left side

the lateral plate to the outer edge of the endoprosthetic head. The necessary minimum length of the femoral neck stump can be predetermined by the correct selection of the height of resection of the femoral neck. Even when selecting the shortest ceramic head, an undesirable and unacceptable increase of leg length of 2 cm or more can result, as the shortest distance from the seating surface of the thrust plate to the outer edge of the head is constant at 43 mm and can be reduced no further. Further shortening would cause the thrust plate to strike the edge of the acetabular cup in cases of extensive hip joint movement. The present dimensions of the prosthesis thus limit its use for slender persons and those of smaller build, which is the case for a major portion of the population of Asia. Particularly for special, anatomically limiting cases, the range of TPPs available has been extended with the size "40 small." This prosthesis version is shortened overall by 7 mm (Figs. 3 and 4).

Endoprosthetics aims to design a foreign body as an artificial joint such that the biomechanical interactions under functional loading conditions corre-

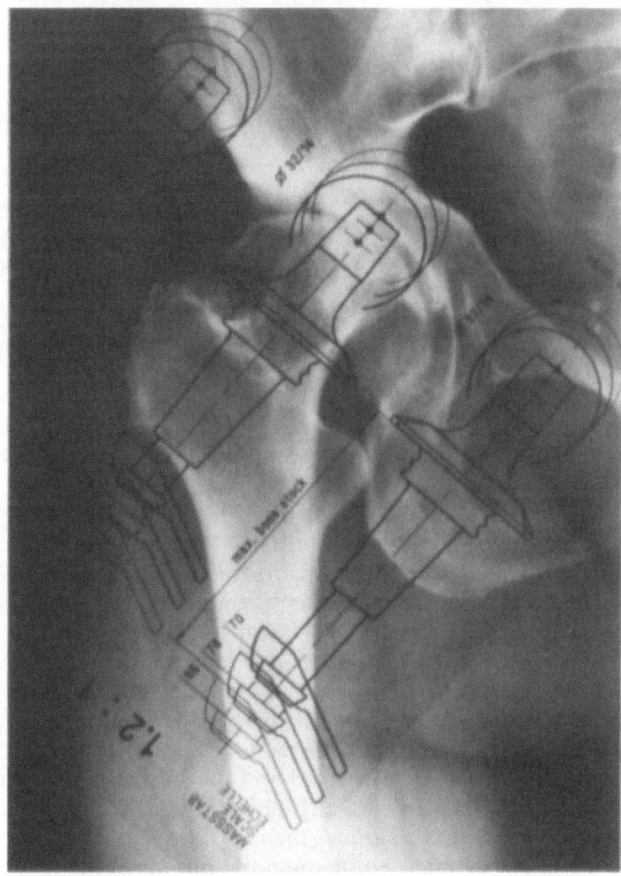

Fig. 3. The preoperative planning shows that the implantation of a TPP even with the shortest bolt is not possible due to the short femoral neck present here

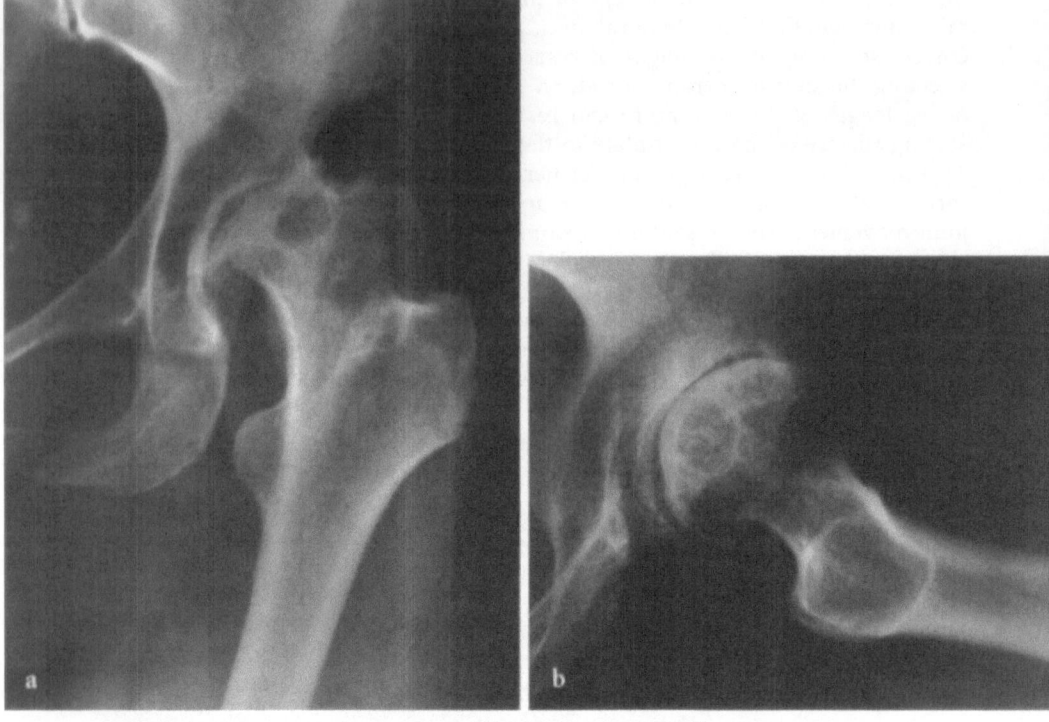

Fig. 4a,b. Functionally valgus femoral neck with residual hip joint dysplasia. Given the short, stocky femoral neck, this represents a borderline case for the implantation of a TPP

spond to nature's original plan, and such that physiological load transfer also actually occurs. Under these conditions the bone must permanently integrate and accept the foreign body. Huggler and Jacob define their requirements for the TPP as follows: "The objective of the thrust plate prosthesis concept is to achieve physiological load transfer from the prosthesis to the proximal femur, in order to avoid loosening through bone resorption as a result of non-physiological loading." This formulation contains two objectives: (a) the possibility of designing a foreign body such that the biomechanical interactions between the implant and the bone under functional loading conditions correspond to nature's original plan, and (b) actually transferring the physiological load. Under these conditions the bone will permanently integrate and accept the foreign body. Physiological load transfer is not possible following resection of the femoral head and part of the femoral neck; however, it is very closely approached with the TPP design. A femoral neck angle between 130° and 135° should be aimed for. The surgical technique for reconstructing the anatomical geometry of the femoral neck is of major significance to the success of the operation, the postoperative behavior, and the prognosis of the TPP. Form deviations in the femoral neck area limit the indication for a TPP (see Figs. 5, 6, 8). Incorrect varus implantation, with nonphysiological load transfer

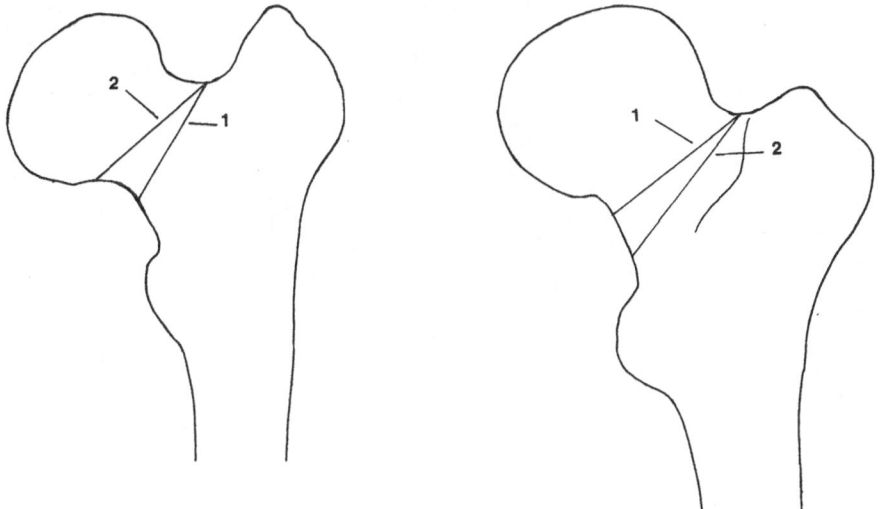

Fig. 5. a Coxa vara. To raise the femoral neck, a flatter osteotomy (*left*) of the femoral neck is needed. *1*, Base of the femoral neck; *2*, necessary corrective osteotomy. **b** Coxa valga. To lower the femoral neck, a steeper osteotomy (*right*) of the femoral neck is needed. *1*, Base of the femoral neck; *2*, necessary corrective osteotomy

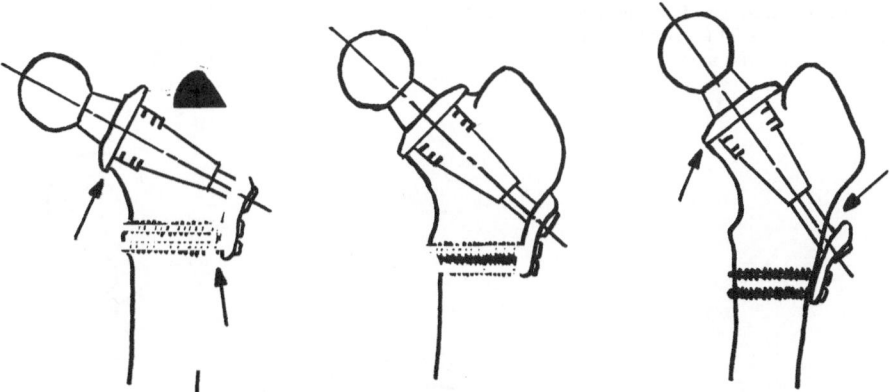

Fig. 6. Limiting indications for the implantation of the TPP with coxa valga and coxa vara. *Left*, steep femoral neck resection for the varus correction of the femoral shaft-neck angle for a preoperative coxa valga condition. Due to this the lateral plate does not touch the femoral cortical bone in its caudal area; *center*, neutral Femoral neck resection with a physiological femoral shaft-neck angle; *right*, more level femoral neck resection in the case of coxa vara. The valgus implantation of the TPP leads to leg lengthening. The lateral plate position is further caudal and cannot fit on the lateral cortical bone in its cranial area. This can present problems during implantation

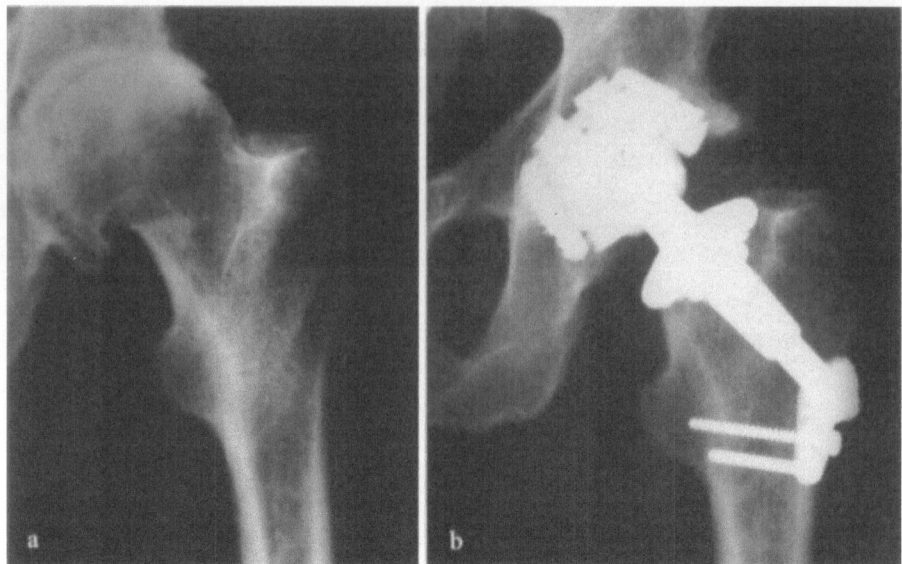

Fig. 7a,b. A 67-year-old man with coxarthrosis on the left side. The valgus axis of the femoral neck was intraoperatively corrected. A femoral shaft-neck angle of 130°–135° is aimed for during implantation of the TPP

Fig. 8a–c. Limiting indications for implantation of the TPP in cases of changed femoral neck antetorsion. **a** Correct implantation of the TPP with physiological femoral neck antetorsion. In cases of increased (**b**) or reduced (**c**) femoral neck antetorsion the TPP cannot be implanted along the axis

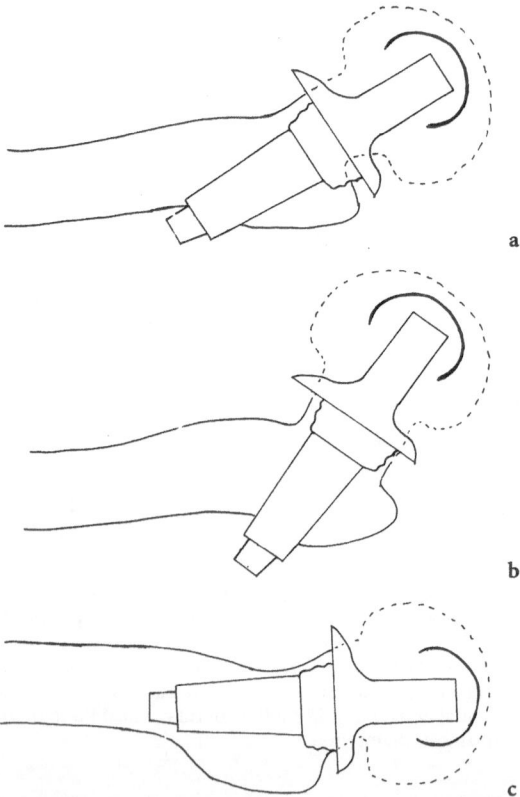

to the coxal femur, may well lead to a higher loosening rate. In cases of coxa vara a valgus adjustment is feasible in principle, and physically desirable, but results in a noticeable lengthening of the leg. Because of the relatively horizontal resection plane (to raise the femoral neck) problems arise with the fit of the lateral plate to the lateral femoral cortical bone. In cases of coxa valga the femoral shaft-neck angle is reduced by a corrective steeper resection of the femoral neck. Corrections of the femoral shaft-neck angle in either varus or valgus directions change the geometry of the femoral neck. This no longer permits the original load transfer to the femur (see Figs. 5–7). The same applies to increased antetorsion, for example, in the case of dysplasia coxarthrosis (see Figs. 8 and 9). Borderline indications can already be recognized as such during

Fig. 9a–c. A 19-year-old man with dysplasia coxarthrosis with Bechterew disease. **a,b** Preoperative radiological status. **c** Postoperative radiological status

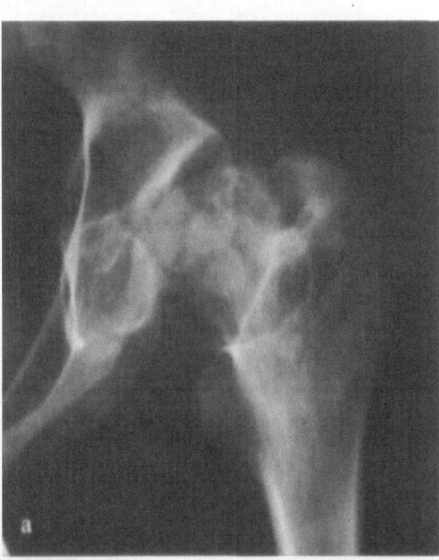

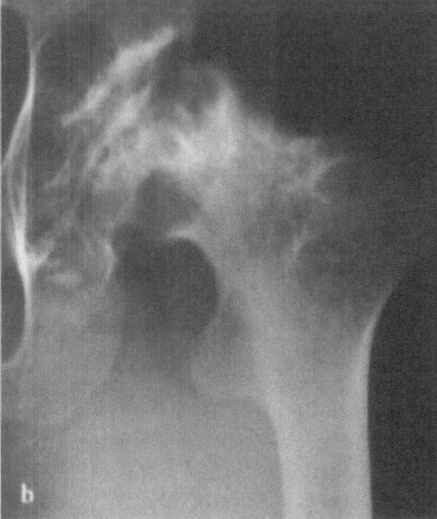

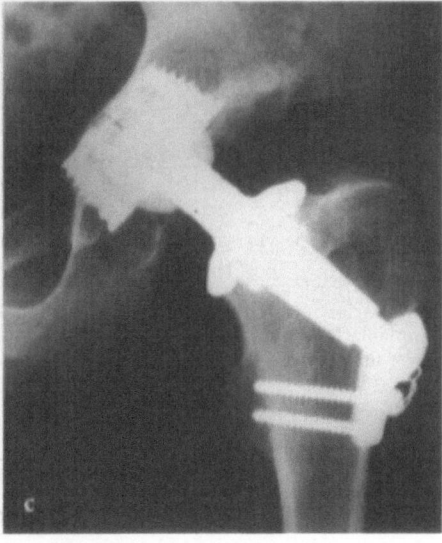

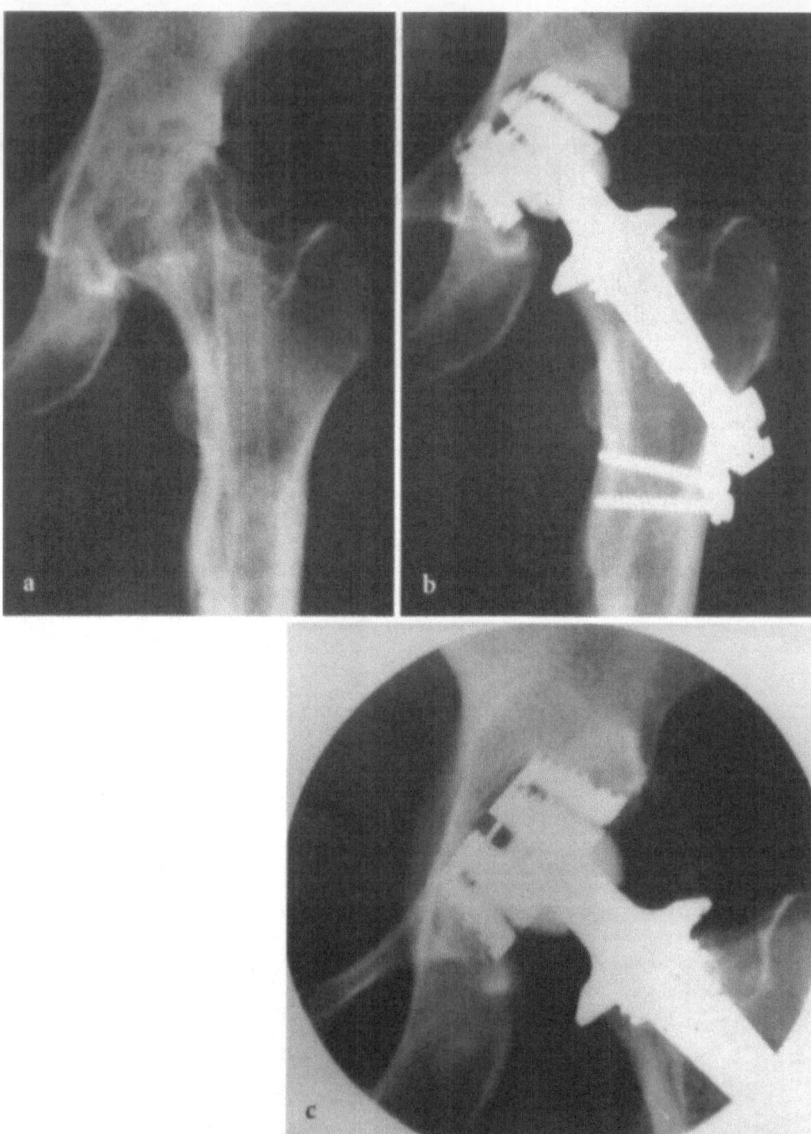

Fig. 10a–c. A 50-year-old woman with post-traumatic coxarthrosis on the left. A femoral shaft fracture was treated osteosynthetically with an intramedullary nail. **a** Preoperative radiological status. **b** Postoperative radiological status. **c** Status on magnifying radiography in the anteroposterior imaging direction. This imaging technique alone allows recognition of incorrect implantations and insufficient areas of contact. In the craniolateral area, a seam can be seen to have formed where the TPP fits on the femoral neck stump

the preoperative planning phase. If, however, it is determined intraoperatively that, contrary to the preoperative drawing, the previously noted anatomical peculiarities would prevent successful implantation, it is then recommended to change to a conventional type of endoprosthesis. Postoperatively the femoral

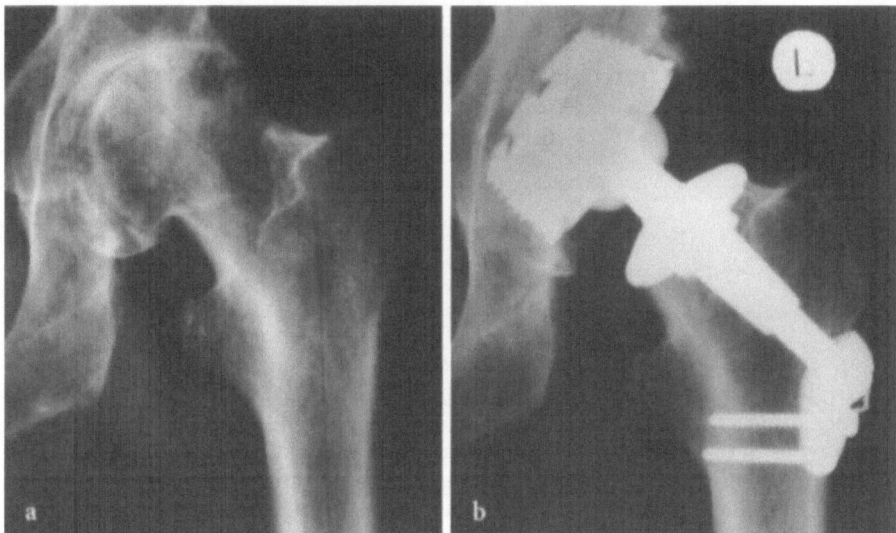

Fig. 11a,b. Preoperative (a) and postoperative (b) radiological status of a TPP implanted along the axis in a 64-year-old patient with coxarthrosis on the left

shaft-neck angle and the assessment of the seating of the endoprosthesis in the area of the femoral neck stump are decisive in the radiological follow-up examination. For this the femoral neck stump is assessed using magnifying radiography in the anteroposterior imaging direction (see Fig. 10c). This imaging technique alone, using correct po-sitioning of the patient, is suitable for judging the seating of the TPP. The TPP represents, when taking account of the contraindications, a good alternative to cement-free standard total hip endoprosthetics. Follow-up treatment corresponds to that for cement-free hip joint alloarthroplasty (Fig. 11).

To summarize, limiting indications for the implantation of a TPP are as follows.

- Anatomically relevant contraindications
  - Short femoral neck
  - Small femoral neck diameter
  - Coxa valga with a femoral shaft-neck angle greater than 140°
  - Coxa vara with a femoral shaft-neck angle below 120°
  - Severe femoral neck antetorsion
- General contraindications
  - Osteoporosis
  - Osteomalacia
  - Alcohol abuse
  - Continuous corticosteroid medication
  - Compensated kidney insufficiency or dialysis
  - Partial loading for 6 weeks not feasible.

CHAPTER 11

Our Experience with the Thrust Plate Prosthesis

J.I. ABAD RICO

Conventional cemented total hip prostheses in young patients show radio-logical and clinical signs of loosening in 70% of cases after 10 years [1–3]. Better long-term results are obtained, however, in elderly patients. Although new types of prostheses with better anchorage have improved results, the long-term integration of prostheses in the host bone still raises problems. The search for more physiological stressing of the femur led to the metaphyseal type of anchorage, the best example of which is the thrust plate prosthesis (TPP). Apart from the biomechanical rationale, this prosthesis allows preservation of bone stock and unimpaired vascularization. It can also easily be replaced by conventional stem prosthesis if this is required. Its design, material, and surface finish are optimal (see Chap. 2, this volume).

From 1991 to July 1994 we implanted 27 TPPs in as many patients, with various hip conditions. There were 20 men and 7 women. The mean age among men was 33.4 years (range 23–61) and that among women 43.3 years (range 22–60). The first 17 patients received the TPP of the second series and the remaining 10 that of the third series. The indications were limited to severely disabling conditions in the following affections:

- Primary osteoarthritis   6
- Secondary osteoarthritis
  - Posttraumatic   4
  - Dysplastic   3
  - Synovial chondromatosis   1
- Idiopathic femoral head necrosis   7
- Secondary femoral head necrosis
  - Posttraumatic   1
  - Corticotherapy   2
  - Alcohol/drugs   3

Of these 27 patients only the first 17, who were operated on before April 1993, were followed-up until 1994; the minimum follow-up time was 15 months in 7 patients, 2 years in 8, and 3 years in 2. The results were rated as good or very good in 13 patients, which means no pain, no limp, and unrestricted daily activity. Their mean Harris hip score was 91. These excellent results were correlated with the subjective opinion of the patients. In two patients there was a leg lengthening of 1.5–2 cm on the operated side which led to sporadic inguinal pain and limp. In these two cases the results were rated as bad. One patient died due to cardiovascular insufficiency and an exacerbation of a lupus

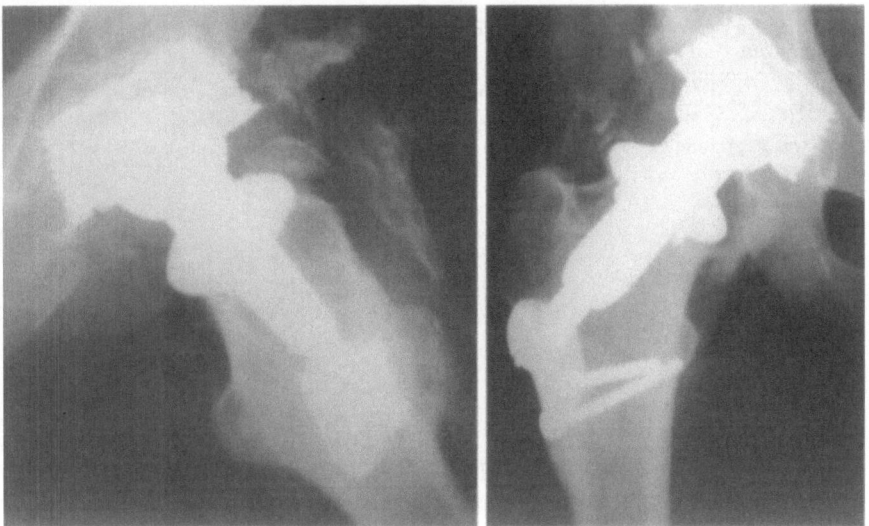

a   b

Fig. 1a,b. Two patients with periarticular ossifications of different extent. There is no impairment of the excellent clinical result

erythematosis condition. Three patients had moderate periarticular ossifications without functional impairment (Fig. 1).

One complication in a 22-year-old woman should be mentioned because it shows in a case of a deep infection that the TPP permits successful and rapid management. The woman was operated on in September 1992 due to secondary osteoarthritis (hip dysplasia). At the time of a follow-up examination 4 months later she complained of local pain. X-rays showed an area of bone resorption medially under the thrust plate. It was decided to inspect the area openly around the lateral plate and to retighten the central bolt. The subsequent local inspection revealed inflammatory tissue with *Pseudomonas aer-*

Fig. 2a

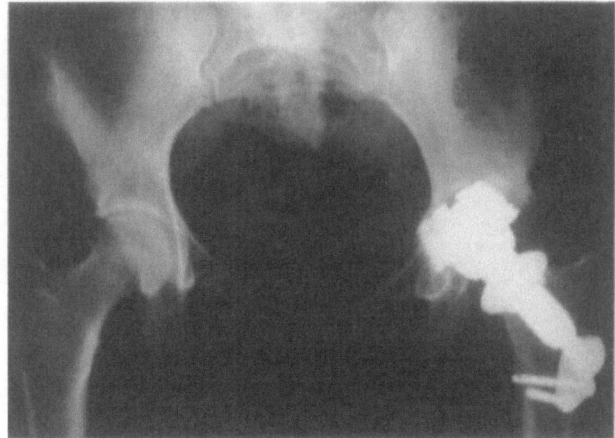

Fig. 2. a As a result of hip dysplasia, a TPP was implanted in a 22-year-old patient. **b** 12 months postoperatively, localized bone resorption in the area of the calcar under the thrust plate is visible after the infection was overcome

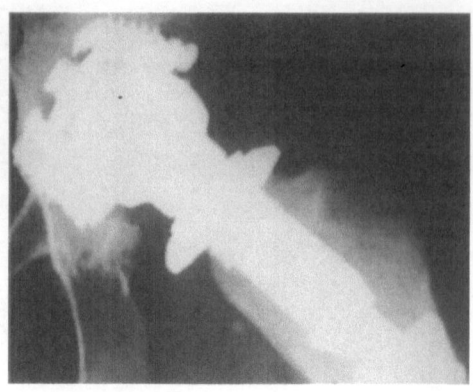

b

uginosa (which was identified in corresponding cultures). Local suction drainage and excision of the infected area were effective (Fig. 2).

In spite of a thorough preoperative planning we encountered technical problems in some cases during the implantation of a TPP. In two patients it was impossible to insert the TPP because it was too large. The thrust plate therefore failed to exert any pressure on the neck stump. In both patients we changed to a conventional stem prosthesis during the operation. In a similar case a bone graft obtained from the resected femoral head was placed under the lateral plate so as to compensate for the large size of the TPP (Fig. 3). Once the TPP was also too voluminous for the patient but was left in place although the thrust plate was probably not seated properly on the femoral stump. The patient was advised to relieve the hip from weight-bearing for an additional

Fig. 3. A bone graft from the femoral neck was placed under the lateral plate to adapt the TPP to the short bone. Two months postoperatively, the bone graft was integrated

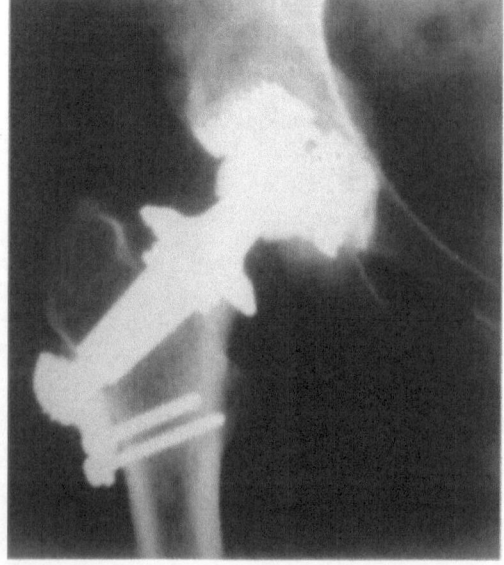

Fig. 4. The femoral neck was too short for the TPP. As a consequence, the thrust plate could not be seated properly on the femoral stump. Nevertheless, the TPP is stable after 8 months with an excellent functional result

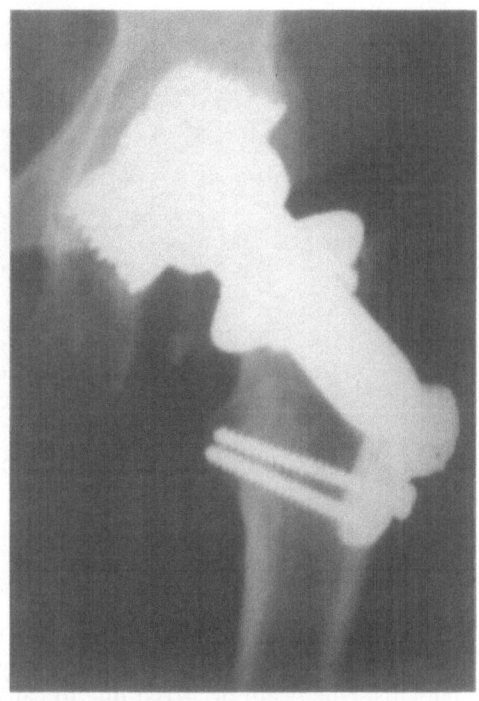

4 weeks (Fig. 4). The results were rated in both patients as "excellent" at the time of follow-up.

In still another patient the femoral neck stump was split when the thrust plate was driven in, which also showed that the size of the TPPs then available was too large for the average size of patients' bone in our geographical area. The fracture of the femoral neck consolidated uneventfully, and the TPP remained stable (Fig. 5). With the availability of a smaller size (40 S) these complications have no longer occurred. Another argument in favor of smaller sizes of the TPP is reflected by the fact that the 86-mm bolt was never used, and the 78-mm bolt in only two patients. The 40-mm thrust plate was implanted in all but two patients, where the 44-mm thrust plate seemed more suitable.

The lateral approach of Bauer seems less harmful to the pelvitrochanteric muscles than the Watson-Jones incision. A proximal and distal elongation of the incision is always possible.

In 1994 we extended the indications to typical osteoarthritic conditions in elderly patients, provided that the host bone exhibits good mineralization, and the general health condition is such that long life can be expected. The indications for implantation in the elderly do not differ from those in younger age groups, although the follow-up time is still insufficient to draw any definite conclusions.

Apart from one infection, all complications were due to the discrepancy between the size of the then available TPP and the size of the average femur in our Spanish population.

Fig. 5. The femoral neck was split when the TPP was driven home. The fracture consolidated uneventfully

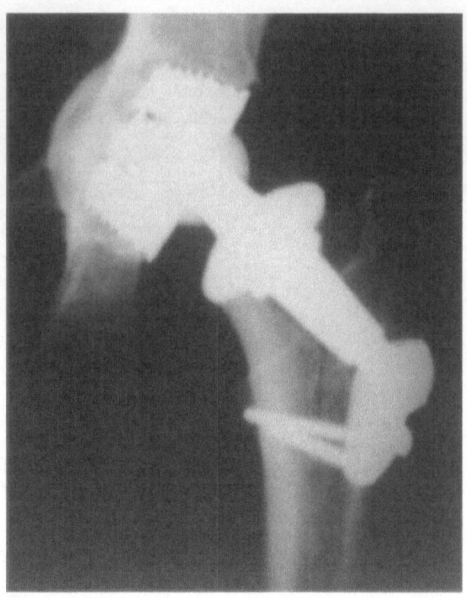

In the initial series of 17 patients, taking into account the phenomenon of the "learning curve," we obtained highly satisfactory results in 76.5% of our patients. One death occurred due to causes unrelated to the hip.

The TPP has proved in our experience to be an excellent prosthesis for the hip, especially in young patients. The short-term results obtained so far and the possibilities of easy change to any conventional prosthesis if this is required at a later date makes this prosthesis particularly interesting. The TPP requires careful surgical technique. Technical errors often lead to failure of the final result.

References

1. Chandler HP, Reineck FT, Wixson RL, McCarthy JC (1981) Total hip replacement in patients younger than thirty years old. J Bone Joint Surg Am 63: 1426–1434
2. Collis DK (1991) Long-term (12–18 yr) follow-up study of cemented total hip replacement in patients who were less than fifty years old. A follow-up note. J Bone Joint Surg Am 73: 593–597
3. Dorr LD, Luckett M, Conaty JP (1990) Total hip arthroplasties younger than 45 years. A 9–10 yr. follow-up study. Clin Orthop 260: 215–219

CHAPTER 12

Chemical Reactions at Titanium Surfaces

M. Schmidt

Introduction

Titanium and its alloys are primarily used in engineering where light weight, high strength and corrosion resistance are required. Their special applicability for cementless implants is due to the superior biocompatibility of these metals. Local and systemic reactions to titanium or titanium alloys used in medicine are basically impossible. This can be shown by the use of physical and chemical principles.

Clinical Observations

Titanium implants with firm primary fixation achieve long-term fixation by osseointegration. Healthy and newly formed bone cells grow onto the titanium surface without intermediate connective tissue. The adhesion of the bone to the surface is very strong and may exceed the normal bone strength. For this to occur, in contrast to implants in CoCrMo alloys for cementless fixation, the surface only needs to exhibit a microstructure with dimensions in the macrometer range. No difference is found between the cellular ongrowth behaviour of pure titanium and its alloys, which are commonly used in medicine.

Titanium, especially the titanium surface, has properties which are not provided by any other metallic biomaterial. This becomes clear when considering the physical and chemical properties of titanium.

Properties

Occurrence

Titanium is the tenth most frequently occurring element in the earth's crust (0.43% by weight). It usually occurs finely distributed in various compounds and seldom in larger deposits. Titanium is therefore quite a common element and is also present in food.

Corrosion Resistance

The surface of the reactive base metal titanium always oxidizes to titanium dioxide (TiO_2). This naturally occurring oxide layer has a thickness of several nanometers and protects the underlying metal very effectively against further corrosive attack. This gives titanium and its alloys a corrosion resistance similar to platinum.

Hydroxylation

The surface layer of TiO_2 is, however, not chemically stable. There is a strong imbalance between the positive titanium cations and the negative oxygen anions, due to the fact that the necessary bonding partners at the surface are missing. The TiO_2 surface achieves a stable, more suitable energy condition by hydroxylation, i.e. by the dissociative adsorption of water molecules from atmospheric water vapour. Two different OH groups are formed on the TiO_2 surface (Fig. 1). The single-coordinated OH groups of basic character are adsorbed by the Ti cations and can be replaced in an acidic environment by other anions. In a basic environment, the proton of the double-coordinated acidic OH groups can be replaced by other cations.

All surface reactions of titanium and its alloys are determined by the natural oxide layer with the hydroxyl groups. The hydroxyl groups hide the underlying layers of TiO_2 and metallic titanium and determine the chemical relationships with the mineralized bone.

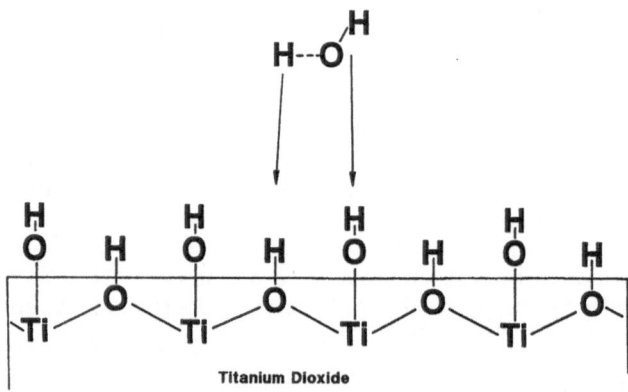

Fig. 1. Very simplified representation of the upper molecular layer of titanium dioxide. As a result of hydroxylation, i.e. the dissociative adsorption of water molecules, a layer of two different OH groups forms. The OH group on the Ti cation is basic and can be replaced by other anions in an acidic environment. The OH group formed at the O anion at the surface is acidic due to dissociation of the proton. In a basic environment, it can be replaced by other cations. The hydroxylation is part of the natural oxidized titanium surface

Solubility

The oxide present on the titanium surface has a very low solubility under biological conditions. A concentration of very few macromoles per litre are sufficient to cause saturation of an aqueous solution with titanium compounds. Additionally, these $Ti(OH)_4(aq)$ aqueous compounds are not ionic, but neutral. Because of their chemical inactivity, they do not interfere with metabolic processes.

Surface Reactions

It is known that many substances are adsorbed onto the oxidized and hydroxylated titanium surface and that the chemical bond between the adsorbate and the surface can be quite strong. Various amino acids belong to the substances which bond very firmly to the surface (Fig. 2). Because amino acids form the basic building blocks of many biological materials and because they significantly determine their boundary surface reactions, it can be assumed that similar reactions will occur around the implant. A layer of autologous molecules must therefore form on the surface of an implant within a very short time.

Biological Reactions to Titanium

The behaviour of titanium in vivo can be easily determined on the basis of the reactive behaviour described above.

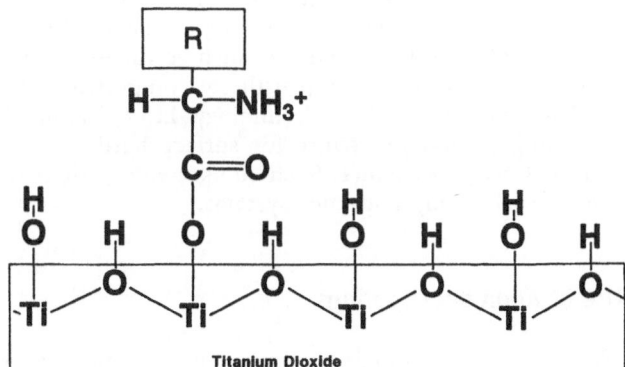

Fig. 2. Very simplified representation of the adsorption of an α-amino acid at the natural (oxidized and hydroxylated) titanium surface. Reactions of this type lead to a strong chemical bonding. This occurs in an acidic aqueous solution by exchange of the basic OH group for the carboxyl group of the amino acid. Other adsorption reactions, e.g. via hydrogen links, are also possible, but lead to weaker chemical bonds

Situation Without an Implant

On account of its frequent occurrence, titanium is continuously being absorbed in small amounts through the digestive tract and is then excreted. The low solubility of titanium compounds ensures that the conditions in the body ensure a saturated solution with respect to titanium. The maximum possible titanium quantity is therefore always present in the body (about 0.2 mmol). Titanium hydrolysis products are therefore not something foreign to the body.

Situation with an Implant

A titanium implant changes nothing in the environment already present, because the surrounding liquid is already saturated with titanium compounds. Under these conditions, further corrosive attack on the implant or allergic reactions to titanium are therefore basically impossible.

Titanium wear particles are of no concern chemically. Because of their insolubility, they remain in the area of their formation. If, however, the tissue becomes too loaded with titanium particles, foreign body reactions may occur due to the number of particles ("particle disease"). Excessive titanium wear must therefore be avoided at all costs.

Usage

Metals which are in direct contact with living tissue should contain no toxic alloying elements. In addition to pure titanium (Protasul-Ti), the forged alloy Ti-6Al-7Nb (Protasul-100) is preferred for the fixation components of cementless Sulzer prosthesis systems. This alloy was developed by Sulzer in the 1980s with the objective of providing a biocompatible high-performance titanium alloy but without elements such as vanadium, which has been found in vitro to be cytotoxic. For prosthesis components articulating against polyethylene, Sulzer Medical Technology Ltd. developed the oxygen-diffusion hardening (ODH) procedure for surface hardening to provide Protasul-100 with high wear resistance. Such components (Tribosul-ODH) are presently in use for various hip and knee systems.

Use of Additional Coatings

Hydroxyapatite or bioglass coatings of cementless titanium implants continue to be promoted. Claims, for example, that these are "bioactive" or even "osteogenetic" indicate the conviction that these coatings achieve more rapid osseointegration or make bony ongrowth possible. From the physicist's point of view, however, such coatings do not make much sense. A few thoughts on this follow:

1. What is in fact ceramic? In the simplest case, it is nothing more than a sintered insoluble metal oxide. Examples of this are the Al_2O_3 and ZrO_2 ceramics used in medicine. With regard to its physical and chemical properties, TiO_2 also belongs to this class of material. Without any addtional effort, titanium implants have a natural TiO_2 bioceramic coating, the quality of which in vivo has been proven by decades of experience. Why, then, should we want to cover it with another coating that is similar but possibly has inferior properties?

2. The promoted coatings are metabolized in the body over time. At some point in time, the bone cells arrive at the original implant surface, and again it needs to be considered whether the implant material and its surface can be osseointegrated. If the cells do not adhere at this point, there is acute risk of implant loosening. A coated implant must therefore be constructed so that it functions safely without coating. Unfortunately, this simple knowledge, which also clearly shows the absurdity of additional coatings, has not yet been fully realized by some manufacturers.

3. Hydroxyapatite coatings do in fact accelerate the ongrowth of bone cells onto the coating, but this in itself is not the whole story. The success or failure of the implant osseointegration depends on the primary stability. Micromotion always prevents bony ongrowth. Where primary stability is present, it is irrelevant whether the biological fixation, giving the prosthesis decades of stability, occurs a few weeks earlier or later.

4. Hydroxyapatite ceramic or bioglass coatings on metallic surfaces are generally only mechanically, and not chemically bonded. This is due both to the properties of the materials involved and to the method of applying the coating using plasma spraying. Thus the danger exists that the coating may disappear from the implant faster than it can be replaced by living bone. The result of this material failure is implant loosening. However, adsorbed body substances are bonded chemically, i.e. safely and permanently, to the titanium surfaces.

5. Even though some sources suggest otherwise, it is not the calcium phosphate coating which brings about osseointegration. Even the most "bioactive" coating is dead material and has decidedly "biopassive" behaviour. Living bone alone osseointegrates metallic implant surfaces if the necessary mechanical and chemical conditions (primary stability, suitable surface structure and materials) are given. Additional coatings actually only hinder the bone cells in this necessary and desirable process.

Despite coatings which require considerable technical effort, the implant is not safer and its indications for use are not increased. The usefulness of bioactive coatings is therefore very doubtful. The user should critically examine whether the relation between effort and benefit is worthwhile. In any case, implants for which osseointegration is claimed based on the coating properties alone, should not be trusted.

Conclusions

Due to the frequency of occurrence of titanium, the body is already saturated with non-toxic titanium corrosion products with low solubility. Systemic reactions following titanium implantation are therefore basically impossible. Local reactions do not occur due to the bioactivity of the surface. The oxidized, hydroxylated titanium with its autologous adsorbate layer is not recognized by the body as a foreign substance.

Titanium and its alloys are ideal materials for implant components which are in direct contact with living tissue. With durable increase in wear resistance using the ODH process, they are also suitable for components which articulate against polyethylene. Additional applied coatings give titanium surfaces no definitive advantages.

General Reading

1. Gerber HW, Moosmann A, Steinemann S (1994) Bioactivity of metals. Tissue tolerance of soluble and solid metal. In: Buchhorn GH, Willert HG (eds) Technical principles. Design and safety of joint implants. Hogrefe and Huber, Göttingen, pp 248–254
2. Schmidt M (1991) Adsorption of Homocysteine on Titanium Surfaces. Helv Phys Acta 64: 900–901
3. Schmidt M (1992) Spezifische Adsorption organischer Moleküle auf oxidiertem Titan: "Bioaktivität" auf molekularem Niveau. Osteologie 1: 222–235
4. Schmidt M, Steinemann SG (1992) XPS studies of amino acids adsorbed on titanium dioxide surfaces. Fresenius J Anal Chem 341: 412–415
5. Semlitsch M, Weber H (1992) Titanlegierung für zementlose Hüftprothesen. In: Hipp E, Gradinger R, Ascherl R (eds) Die zementlose Hüftprothese. Demeter, Gräfelfing, pp 18–26
6. Steinemann SG (1994) Corrosion of implant alloys. In: Buchhorn GH, Willert HG (eds) Technical principles. Design and safety of joint implants. Hogrefe and Huber, Göttingen, pp 168–179
7. Streicher RM, Weber H, Schön R, Semlitsch M (1991) New surface modification for Ti-6AI-7Nb alloy: oxygen diffusion hardening (ODH). Biomaterials 12: 125–129
8. Streicher RM, Weber H, Schon R, Semlitsch MF (1992) Wear resistant couplings for longer lasting articulating total joint replacements. In: Doherty PJ et al (eds) Biomaterial-tissue-Interfaces. Elsevier, Amsterdam, pp 179–186
9. Zweymüller K, Lintner F, Semlitsch M (1988) Biologic fixation of a press-fit titanium hip joint endoprosthesis. Clin Orthop Rel Res 235: 195–206

CHAPTER 13

Material Combinations with Polyethylene and Metasul for Articulating Implants

R.M. STREICHER

Introduction

After a break of 20 years, it is now recognized once more that polymer wear particles, in particular, significantly affect the long-term fixation results of cemented and cementless prostheses through necrosis, osteolysis and subsequent loosening; as a result, interest in implant tribology has now increased again. Compared with the natural joint, the tribological situation in an artificial joint is fundamentally changed by the use of artificial, non-porous materials as articulating surfaces. Given the continuously changing loading and velocity conditions in the body, a lubricating film can only be temporary. Solid body contact between the articulating components of the artificial joint is therefore almost always present, with unavoidable high friction values and material wear. The amount of wear per unit of time is a particularly important factor regarding possible osteolysis; in addition to the chemical composition, the size and morphology of the wear particles are also important [18]. Only a few small particles can be carried away by the patient's peri-articular system, and little or no foreign body reactions are likely. The objective of improvements in materials and their combination as articulating implant components must therefore be directed towards the reduction of the number of wear particles, if possible with a simultaneous reduction of friction.

Tribology

Tribology is the science of friction, lubrication and wear processes that not only depend on the system, but also on specific material properties. Friction and lubrication conditions in a tribosystem can generally be divided into two states. With *fluid film lubrication*, as is the case in the healthy human joint, the two solid bodies are completely separated by an intermediate fluid. With *dry or boundary lubrication*, on the other hand, the surfaces of the articulating bodies are in direct contact with each other. The term *mixed lubrication*, as in the case of a diseased joint or an artificial joint, refers to the area of fluid film lubrication in which the intermediate fluid can only partially separate the two bodies.

The tribological system in a human joint consists of two solid bodies (bone), each of which is covered with a porous, elastic layer (cartilage). Between and around them is the structurally viscous synovial lubricating fluid. In healthy patients, this aqueous dialysate of blood plasma with proteins, salts and a high molecular weight protein (hyaluronic acid) more or less completely separates the two solid bodies, depending on cartilage function. The tribosystem is sealed within an impermeable membrane (capsule). The contact-free articulation in the natural joint results in low friction and under normal conditions is wear-free, with a low friction coefficient of less than 0.025 [7]. In the case of rheumatic disease of the joint, for example, the reduced lubricating capacity of the synovia, among other factors, no longer ensures fluid film lubrication, and severe wear of the joint surfaces can occur. The increased friction values and the associated pain then lead in the long term to the necessity of replacing the affected joint with an artificial one.

A selection of clinically successful material combinations for prosthesis articulating surfaces and their long-term results for hip endoprostheses are shown in Fig. 1. Whereas for these implants several metallic and ceramic materials are suitable, knee prostheses only permit the use of ultra-high molecular weight polyethylene (UHMWPE) with CoCrMo alloy.

Since the replacement of the metal/metal combination in the 1960s, the standard material combination for artificial hip joints is UHMWPE cups with austenitic steel or CoCrMo alloy ball heads. The combinations are used in diameters of 22, 26, 28, 32 and 37 mm and have a mean linear wear rate of 0.05–0.25 mm/year. Attempts to strengthen the polyethylene or to replace this material with other polymers have so far been unsuccessful. However, the substitution of metallic ball heads of 32 mm by Al_2O_3 ceramic heads gave reduced UHMWPE wear values of less than 0.13 mm/year [20]. Ceramic heads of the same diameter, when articulating against ceramic, gave a very low wear rate of 8 µm/year if the hip prosthesis was ideally positioned [3]. If the cup is implanted steeply, however (>50°), excessive edge pressure can result in catastrophic wear [4]. Investigation of explanted metal/metal hip prostheses with

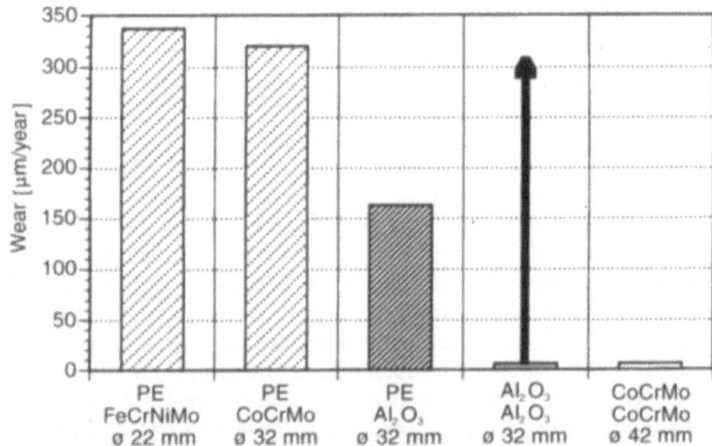

Fig. 1. Wear rates of various material combinations in vivo. *PE*, polyethylene

long implantation times showed that this particular material combination has wear rates of only very few micrometres per year [8], with a correspondingly low wear-particle load on the peri-articular tissue.

Tribological Investigations

Before new materials and designs are put to clinical studies, their tribological behaviour must first be investigated in the laboratory. A comparison of various test methods is shown in Table 1. In order to ensure that the conditions for tribological investigations are as realistic as possible and to allow comparison between different laboratories, several guidelines and standards have been prepared: e.g. ISO TR 9325 and 9326, ASTM F 732. For these investigations, a class 10 000 air-conditioned clean-room with class 100 (particles/m^3) laminar air flow boxes placed directly over the individual testing equipment was set up as the tribology laboratory in order to eliminate any possible influence on the results due to contamination from the surrounding air. In addition, the fluid medium for all the tests is sterile filtered using a 0.2-μm membrane filter, with the testing area around each testing chamber covered. The fluid medium for all standard tests is a mixture of Ringer's solution with 30% calf serum, buffered to pH 7.2, with the proportions of proteins and mineral salts corresponding to synovia [19].

Laboratory Testing Using Pin-on-Disk Models

Laboratory testing using pin-on-disk models can provide a large number of results in a short time using relatively simple testing equipment and little

Table 1. Tribological testing phases

Method	Advantages/Disadvantages
Model test (pin-on-disk)	Loading different from in vivo
	Fast (7 days), economical
	Simple, cheap machines
	Only general information
Model test with implants (pendulum)	More similar loading situation
	Fast (minutes)
	General information
	Only friction values
Simulator test	Close approximation to physiological loading
	Long testing time (several months)
	Expensive, sophisticated machines
	Complex
	Specific information
Clinical investigation	Physiological loading
	Difficult and expensive study
	Long testing time (years)
	Individual loading differences
	Large variance in
	results

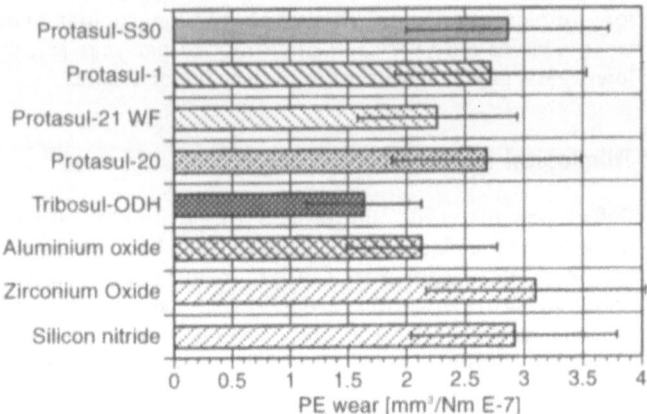

Fig. 2. Comparison of polyethylene (*PE*) wear rates in pin-on-disk tests

effort. The simplification of conditions in vivo, however, affects the relevance of such tests, and the results must only be applied to clinical use with caution and careful interpretation. It is important to take into account the tribosystem with the combination of roughness, wear and friction behaviour together with observations of changes in the articulating surfaces.

Various material combinations were tested in the tribology laboratory in pin-on-disk testing machines (CSEM Tribometer) with disks made of the harder material and pins of UHMWPE. The testing conditions are matched in simplified form to those occurring naturally [11]. Similar to the wear, the friction coefficient is also monitored on a continuous basis using a computer (Macintosh, Labview 3.0). Figure 2 shows the wear results as mean values from at least six tests on pin-on-disk models. The standard deviation of individual results was in the range of 10%–50% of the mean values and is small in comparison with the clinical investigation results.

A clear correlation was found between the roughness of the Protasul-1 CoCrMo alloy disks and polyethylene wear, as is typical for an articulation of two non-polar materials under mixed lubrication conditions. Such a correlation for steel alloys is mentioned in the literature [1]. The roughness of the CoCrMo alloy can be reduced by forging (Protasul-21WF). In laboratory tests, the reduction in size of the hard carbides protruding from the matrix brought about lower polyethylene wear and a lower friction coefficient. The tribological investigation of mirror-finish polished FeCrNiMnMoNbN alloy Protasul-S30 articulating against UHMWPE gave a polyethylene wear rate similar to the CoCrMo alloy, but with a reduced friction coefficient. In all tests using iron- and cobalt-based materials, the surface of the disk was not scratched when articulating against UHMWPE pins.

On the other hand, when using titanium alloys, there was massive titanium and polyethylene wear with associated black discoloration of the test medium. In order to improve these well-known adverse tribological characteristics of a material which is otherwise ideal for cementless implant fixation, various possibilities for surface modification were investigated tribologically. Treatment of the titanium alloy surface using nitrogen ion implantation [9] to a maximum depth of 0.8 μm using this process led to increased UHMWPE wear and proved to be tribologically unstable, even against polyethylene. The use of bone cement instead of polyethylene as the pin material led to rapid abrasion of the treated surface layer. This surface treatment of articulating titanium alloys for implants therefore appears to be unsatisfactory.

Hardening of the titanium surface using oxygen diffusion (Tribosul-ODH [15]) resulted in clearly reduced polyethylene wear, similar to Al_2O_3 ceramic, with low friction and represents a fracture-safe alternative. Due to the excellent wettability of this surface, the fact that its hardness (1200 HV) is three times higher than CoCrMo surfaces, its low modulus of elasticity, which results in lower contact stresses in the polyethylene tibia plateau, and finally the osseo-conductivity of the titanium alloy surface [6], it is especially interesting for the femoral components of knee endoprostheses.

Articulation of aluminium oxide disks (Al_2O_3, ISO 6474) against UHMWPE pins resulted in a reduction in wear and friction values compared with metal disks (although not to the same extent as in vivo). A reduction of UHMWPE wear rate of 30%–75% in vivo compared with metal ball heads has been reported [17, 20], and only 20% was measured in the laboratory. This difference can be explained by the fact that it is not possible to obtain the same surface quality on flat, hard oxide ceramic disks as on the ball heads. The alternative zirconium oxide ceramic (ZrO_2) and silicon nitride (Si_3N_4) gave higher wear and friction values in all cases [16].

Also investigated was the influence of irradiation sterilization on the tribological behaviour of Sulene-PE, which is a highly polymerized medical-grade polyethylene, moulded in a clean-room without additives [13]. The changes occurring in the molecular structure of UHMWPE during sterilization using ionizing radiation can be put to advantage by the use of an inert gas atmosphere during the irradiation process [12]. Polyethylene that is irradiation sterilized in this manner displays an approximately 50% lower wear rate than when sterilized in air, while the friction coefficient remains the same.

Laboratory Tests Using Implants (Pendulum Equipment)

The testing machines used mostly have only one degree of freedom, producing simpler movements and/or loading patterns than in the in vivo situation. An example is the Buchs pendulum testing machine [5], in which the friction characteristics of various material combinations can be investigated.

Because excessive friction moments had been blamed for the loosening of earlier metal/metal hip systems [8], the articulation of various CoCrMo alloys against themselves was tested with various ball head sizes.

Additionally, the reference combinations of Al_2O_3 and CoCrMo ball heads 32 mm in diameter articulating against UHMWPE were tested. The results showed that the 37-mm CoCrMo alloy metal/metal combination had a friction moment 70%–100% higher than the 32-mm-diameter CoCrMo and Al_2O_3

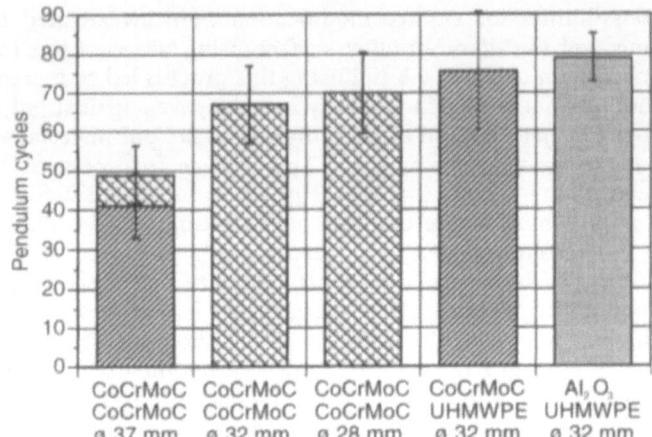

Fig. 3. Comparison of various material combinations in the pendulum test. *UHMWPE*, ultra-high molecular weight polyethylene

combinations with polyethylene. The reduction of the ball diameter of the metal/metal combination to 32 and 28 mm, as well as the use of the CoCrMo forging alloy Protasul-21WF instead of the cast alloy Protasul-1, reduced friction losses in the lubricated condition down to the values of the polymer/metal combination, as shown in Fig. 3. A comparison with prostheses retrieved after clinical use showed close correlation with the friction behaviour values obtained from the pendulum experiment.

Hip and Knee Simulators

Hip and knee simulators employing complicated mechanical systems with loading combinations as in vivo were used to investigate the potentially successful material combinations selected from the simpler tests. The mechanical hip simulators used (Stanmore Mk III [19]) produce a natural loading pattern with an adapted double peak which, in these machines, unlike all others used (e.g. [2]), is applied kinematically with all three degrees of freedom.

Since the results obtained from the pendulum tests showed comparable friction values and the investigations of explants showing wear volume indicated far lower wear of metal/metal combinations compared with polymer/metal or ceramic combinations, the tribological behaviour of CoCrMo combinations of ball heads with different diameters was investigated in detail. In the hip simulator, the metal/metal combination showed the clear effect of the geometry of the contact surfaces, particularly in the smaller head of 28 mm in diameter with correspondingly high surface contact pressures. All combinations tested in the hip simulator had running-in wear in the region of 10–20 μm on each component, during which period the articulation surfaces adjust to each other. With suitable geometric conditions, there was then a transition from running-in wear to a stable low-wear of 2–4 µm/million cycles per component; where geometric conditions were not appropriate, there was heavy wear on both components. The linear wear measured in the simulator for implants with optimum surface machining is practically identical to that measured on explants retrieved after long-term use [14]. In comparison with retrieved implants, however, those from the simulators showed a preferential wear direction with increased groove wear, due to the controlled kinematic conditions. The friction moment measured in the hip simulator for combinations with a ball diameter of 37 mm were 5–7 Nm, 100%–200% higher than for the 32-mm-diameter polymer/metal combinations. With decreasing head diameter and the same nominal clearance, the contact surface with the M_3C_7 block carbides is reduced, hence also the friction resistance. Friction moment values similar to the polymer/metal combination were measured in the pendulum test for metal/metal combinations using ball heads of the CoCrMo forged alloy with reduced roughness, with a smaller diameter of 28 mm and after the clearance within the cup had been optimized. The friction moment and the wear were higher in the running-in period, but stabilized after 0.5–1 million cycles with low friction and wear conditions.

Simulators (Stallforth/Ungethüm [10]) with 60° flexion and implant-specific sliding movement were also used for testing the tribological behaviour of knee endoprostheses. The results of the tests using knee prosthesis models with femoral parts of CoCrMo cast alloy Protasul-1 and forged, oxygen diffusion-hardened titanium alloy Protasul-100 (Tribosul-ODH) combined with tibial plateaux in Sulene-PE showed a good correlation of the UHMWPE wear rate with the results of the model tests. The Tribosul-ODH articulating surface produced significantly less polyethylene wear than that in Protasul-1, as shown in Fig. 4. Similarly to explanted knee prostheses of similar design, the CoCrMo femoral part showed scratches in the articulating direction of the prosthesis

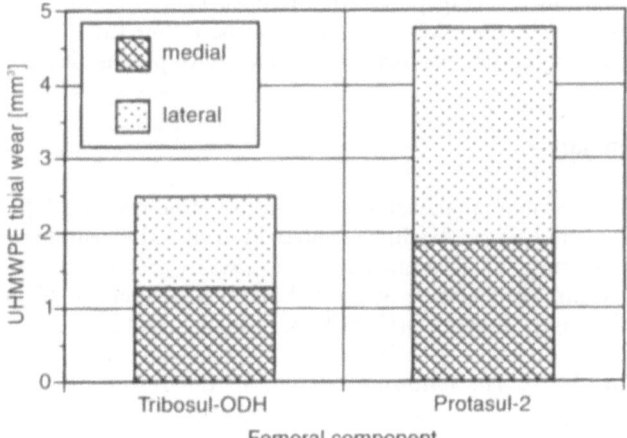

Fig. 4. Comparison of polyethylene wear rates in the knee simulator. *UHMWPE*, ultra-high molecular weight polyethylene

after the test, which in some cases could be traced to exposed catalyst residue in the UHMWPE. The hardened titanium surfaces, especially the Tribosul-ODH femoral part, showed very few scratches, even after several million cycles.

Clinical Investigation

This investigation is highly relevant, although the results may vary significantly according to the clinic at which the investigation is performed and the assessment method. Measurements from radiographs may provide different results, depending on the positioning and assessment methods used, and are only meaningful where there are high wear rates. Wear values from explants are always higher than measurements from radiographs due to the negative selection process. The mean linear wear rate of explanted UHMWPE hip-joint cups in combination with 32-mm-diameter CoCrMo alloy ball heads for 10 years in vivo was 0.23 mm/year. Explants from male patients showed a 25% higher wear rate. Explanted cups with three-body wear caused by bone cement particles showed a wear rate increase of more than 50%, but this was no longer significant for cups that had been implanted for more than 10 years. Patient weight, age at operation and the angle of main loading showed no correlation with the PE wear rate on the investigated implants, unlike the length of time implanted. As had already been determined in laboratory tests, the generation of wear particles is directly proportional to the amount of movement which has occurred and thus also to patient activity.

Wear measurements on explanted all-metal prostheses of various designs with diameters of 35–42 mm and implantation times of up to 25 years showed yearly wear rates of 0.4–0.8 μm on each component, regardless of prosthesis type. The visual appearance of the articulating surfaces improved over time, because the loading marks from the running-in of the ball head in the cup were continuously being polished. In those very few metal/metal prostheses with higher wear, the cause was found to be either the deformation of thin-walled cups or tolerance problems associated with production methods in those days.

Summary

Before a new material or design for the articulating components of endoprostheses can be investigated in trials, the tribological behaviour of the articulating surfaces must be examined in the laboratory. In order to achieve an optimum overview of the tribological behaviour of material combinations and designs, it is important, if possible, to select not just one test method but to proceed stepwise with increasing degrees of complexity before proceeding to clinical use. The clinical relevance of the results obtained should always be assessed by comparison with known negative and positive reference values.

Laboratory tests indicated that UHMWPE is basically a good articulation partner for various metal and ceramic materials. The Sulene-PE grade of moulded UHMWPE, produced under optimized manufacturing conditions, has significantly lower wear values following irradiation sterilization in inert gas.

The combination of UHMWPE with CoCrMo alloys of lower surface roughness and especially with high-grade Al_2O_3 ceramic resulted in even lower wear values and in lower friction. Although alternative ceramics are stronger and tougher, they exhibit higher polyethylene wear in the pin-on-disk test. The surface hardening of titanium alloy using ion implantation also produced no tribological advantages. However, the Tribosul-ODH surface, produced by oxygen diffusion hardening, exhibited both much lower polyethylene wear and significantly less friction in the pin-on-disk test and in the knee simulator. The high surface hardness, the osseoconductivity of the coarse blasted titanium alloy for fixation and the low modulus of elasticity would appear to make the use of Tribosul-ODH ideal, especially for knee endoprostheses articulating against UHMWPE.

Investigation of the metal/metal combination (Metasul) in various tribological tests showed the potential of the CoCrMo forged alloy Protasul-21WF with reduced surface roughness and increased strength for articulations of hip endoprostheses. If the clearance between ball head and cup has been correctly selected and manufactured, especially in the case of heads with smaller diameters, the running-in period is followed by a stable phase with friction values comparable to those obtained with combinations employing polyethylene, but with a wear rate reduced by several orders of magnitude. Use of the Metasul technology in such implants results in a reduction in the risk of late particle-induced loosening of hip prostheses.

References

1. Cooper JR, Dowson D, Fisher J (1993) The effect of transfer film and surface roughness on the wear of lubricated UHMWPE. Clin Mat 14: 295–302
2. McKellop HA, Clarke IC (1984) Evolution and evaluation of materials screening machines and joint simulators in predicting in vivo wear phenomena. In: Ducheyne P, Hasting GW (eds) Functional behavior of orthopedic biomaterials, vol II: applications. CRC, Boca Raton, pp 51–85
3. Mittelmeier H, Heisel J (1990) Fifteen years of experience with ceramic hip prostheses. In: Aldinger G, Sell S, Beyer A (eds) Noncemented total hip replacement. Thieme, Stuttgart, pp 142–150
4. Plitz W, Hoss H-U (1980) Untersuchungen zum Verschleimechanismus bei revidierten Hüftendoprothesen mit Gleitflächen aus Al_2O_3 -Keramik. Biomed Tech 25: 165–168
5. Ruesch R, Thöny C (1981) Reibungsversuche an künstlichen Hüftgelenken. Diplomarbeit, Technikum Buchs
6. Schmidt M (1992) Spezifische Adsorption organischer Moleküle auf oxidiertem Titan: "Bioaktivität" auf molekularem Niveau. Osteologie 174: 222–235
7. Schurz J (1983) Biorheologie. Probleme und Ergebnisse in der Medizin. Naturwissenschaften 70: 602–608
8. Semlitsch MF, Streicher RM, Weber H (1989) Verschleiverhalten von Pfannen und Kugeln aus CoCrMo-Gulegierung bei langzeitig implantierten Ganzmetall-Hüftprothesen. Orthopädie 18: 36–41
9. Sioshansi P, Oliver RW, Matthews FD (1985) Wear improvement of surgical alloys by ion implantation. J Vac Sci Tech A3: 2670–2674

10. Stallforth H, Ungethüm M (1978) Die tribologische Testung von Knieendoprothesen. Biomed Techn 23/12: 295–304
11. Streicher RM (1989) Tribologie in der Medizin: Prüfung und Optimierung von Materialpaarungen für die Endoprothetik. Neuere Biomaterialien für die Endoprothetik, Berlin, pp 20–39 (Praxis-Forum 19)
12. Streicher RM (1989) Investigation on sterilization and modification of HMW-Polyethylenes by ionizing irradiation. Beta Gamma 1/89: 34–43
13. Streicher RM (1993) UHMW-Polyethylen als Werkstoff für artikulierende Komponenten von Gelenkendoprothesen. Biomed Techn 38/12: 303–313
14. Streicher RM, Schön R, Semlitsch M (1990) Untersuchung des tribologischen Verhaltens von Metall/Metall-Kombinationen für künstliche Hüftgelenke. Biomed Techn 35/5: 107–111
15. Streicher RM, Weber H, Schön R, Semlitsch M (1991) New surface modification for Ti-6Al-7Nb alloy: Oxygen Diffusion Hardening (ODH). Biomaterials 12: 125–129
16. Streicher RM, Semlitsch M, Schön R (1991) Ceramic surfaces as wear partners for polyethylene. In: Bonfield W, Hastings GW, Tanner KE (eds) Bioceramics, vol 4. Butterworth-Heinemann, Oxford, pp 9–16
17. Weber BG (1981) Total hip replacement: rotating versus fixed and metal against ceramic heads. In: Salvati E (ed) The hip. Mosby, St Louis, pp 264–275
18. Willert H-G, Semlitsch MF (1977) Reactions of the articular capsule to wear products of artificial joint prostheses. J Biomed Mat Res 11: 157–164
19. Wright KWJ (1982) Friction and wear of materials and joint replacement prostheses. In: Williams DF (ed) Biocompatibility of orthopedic implants, vol I. CRC, Boca Raton, pp 141–195
20. Zichner LP, Willert H-G (1992) Comparison of alumina-polyethylene and metal-polyethylene in clinical trials. Clin Orth Rel Res 282: 86–94